Also by Pete Magill

Build Your Running Body
(with Thomas Schwartz and Melissa Breyer)

THE BORN AGAIN RUNNER

A Guide to Overcoming Excuses, Injuries,
and Other Obstacles—for New
and Returning Runners

PETE MAGILL

Photographs by Diana Hernandez

THE EXPERIMENT

NEW YORK

The Experiment, LLC
220 East 23rd Street, Suite 301
New York, NY 10010-4674
www.theexperimentpublishing.com

This book is not intended as a substitute for the medical advice of physicians or other clinicians. Readers should consult with a physician, dietitian, or other health care professional before beginning or making any changes to a diet, exercise, or health program. The authors and publisher expressly disclaim responsibility for any liability, loss, or risk—personal or otherwise—which is incurred, directly or indirectly, as a consequence of the use and application of any of the contents of this book.

Neither this book nor any opinion or recommendation expressed by the author within the book is supported or endorsed by the owner of any trademark that may be visible on any running shoe or any other product that appears in any photo. In one instance, the author recommends a specific branded product that is displayed in the accompanying photo. Otherwise, any product whose brand name is visible is portrayed solely to illustrate the text.

The Experiment's books are available at special discounts when purchased in bulk for premiums and sales promotions as well as for fundraising or educational use. For details, contact us at info@theexperimentpublishing.com.

Library of Congress Cataloging-in-Publication Data

Names: Magill, Pete.
Title: The born again runner : a guide to overcoming excuses, injuries, and
  other obstacles for new and returning runners / Pete Magill ; photographs
  by Diana Hernandez.
Description: New York : The Experiment, LLC, [2016] | "Distributed by Workman
  Publishing Company, Inc."--T.p. verso.
Identifiers: LCCN 2016007856 (print) | LCCN 2016022975 (ebook) | ISBN
  9781615193110 (Paperback) | ISBN 9781615193127 (Ebook)
Subjects: LCSH: Running--Training--Handbooks, manuals, etc. |
  Running--Physiological aspects--Handbooks, manuals, etc. | Runners
  (Sports)--Handbooks, manuals, etc.
Classification: LCC GV1061.5 .M236 2016 (print) | LCC GV1061.5 (ebook) | DDC
  613.7/172--dc23
LC record available at https://lccn.loc.gov/2016007856

ISBN 978-1-61519-311-0
Ebook ISBN 978-1-61519-312-7

Cover and text design by Sarah Smith

Manufactured in China
Distributed by Workman Publishing Company, Inc.
Distributed simultaneously in Canada by Thomas Allen and Son Ltd.

First printing August 2016
10 9 8 7 6 5 4 3 2 1

CONTENTS

INTRODUCTION

"Things do not change; we change."
—HENRY DAVID THOREAU

BY ALL RIGHTS, I shouldn't be writing this book.

I should be grossly overweight, plagued with a smoker's hack, tasting last night's whiskey at the back of my throat, and sucking wind from the effort it took to roll my desk chair forward so that my fingers could reach the keyboard.

Or I should be dead.

Dead was the prediction of the emergency room physician who treated me late one night during the winter of 2000. I was thirty-eight years old, recently divorced, fifty pounds overweight, splitting care of my six-year-old son, Sean, with my ex-wife, Jinny, and working around the clock as a struggling Hollywood screenwriter. I was sleeping two to three hours per night. Was living on a diet of junk food, hard liquor, Marlboros, and various amphetamines—only sobering up long enough to attend weekly court-ordered meetings for my various alcohol-related offenses. My physical activity consisted of thrice-weekly outings to local parks with Sean; he'd chase me around playground equipment until my face turned red and I got too dizzy to stand (think Marlon Brando in *The Godfather* just moments before he pitches face-first into the tomato plants). And then one night, alone at home, I did collapse, tumbling unconscious to the floor.

Later that night, at Verdugo Hills Hospital, the ER physician explained that I'd gotten off easy, that I hadn't had a heart attack, stroke, or something more serious. Instead, I was exhausted, overworked, and suffering the predictable effects of massive substance abuse. And then he added, "Of course, at the rate you're going, you won't live to see your son graduate from high school."

Something had to change.

But where to start? Everything about my life was a mess. My workload. My diet. My weight. My sleeping habits. My parental obligations. Not to mention my attempt to manage all of the above with a suspended driver's license, morning shakes, heart arrhythmia, anxiety attacks, and zero friends who weren't headed down the same road, who weren't accelerating toward the same brick wall.

I was overwhelmed. And I'd lost control of my life.

Of course, you didn't open this book to read about me. You opened this book to find relevant, effective, and practical information on starting a running program that works for you. You have your own hurdles to clear. If not, you'd already be running. You have your own bad habits, your own physical shortcomings, your own work problems and health issues and personal foibles. In short, you aren't focused on how I did it, how I crawled out of my rabbit hole and rejoined the world a fitter, happier, and saner person. You need to know how you can do it.

I hear you.

And I want to assure you right now, as we decide whether to step out the door together and follow the path laid out in the chapters ahead, that this book doesn't tell my story—even if that's where it starts, and even if I'll be injecting elements of my story into its pages.

This book tells your story.

It tells the story of your busy life and full schedule. And of the reasons you've procrastinated about starting an exercise program. It addresses weight, health, chronic injury, disability, lack of time, and other issues that might have gotten in your way. It recognizes the anxiety (and even fear) that sometimes holds potential new runners back from taking the first step. And for those of you who simply want a *dos and don'ts* manual, it offers comprehensive instruction for every step of your new program.

This book is a road map for changing yourself—for becoming a runner and achieving the results you associate with that goal (whether that means weight loss, improved health, decreased stress, simply having fun, or finishing the Boston Marathon).

And that's where my story comes into play, because before you'll believe me when I say *you will succeed*, you need to know that I succeeded, that like the mythical phoenix rising from the ashes, I conjured a practicing runner from the mess I'd made of my life.

The ER physician's warning was a wake-up call. But my takeaway wasn't a fear of impending death. Dying was an abstract concept, and one that even the physician had admitted lay in a semi-distant and nebulous future. My motivation was far more immediate: I didn't want to continue living the way that I had. The problem was figuring out an escape plan. Too much was wrong with my life—and had been for a long, long time.

I'd started drinking at age thirteen, on the basketball courts at Foothill Intermediate School. I'd meet a couple friends during lunch, and we'd mix vodka or gin or whiskey with Coca-Cola that we'd purchased in the cafeteria. A painfully shy, one-hundred-pound weakling, I gained confidence from alcohol during a time when I was pretty much terrified of every other kid in the school. My behavior only got worse in high school. Even as I made the varsity cross country team my freshman year, earning a status upgrade among my classmates, I added cigarettes and drugs to my ever-increasing alcohol consumption. After high school, I hitchhiked around the USA and traveled Europe by train, managing to get blackout drunk in multiple major cities on both continents. And then I tried college, at UC Berkeley, USC, Glendale Community College, and Cal State L.A. I tried running at each. And I tried studying at each. But it didn't work out. Every time, partying eventually won the day. So I bought a cheap around-the-world airline ticket (a single-fare ticket that allowed me to fly unlimited legs and miles to anywhere in the world, as long as I kept moving in a single direction) and headed west. If I couldn't manage my life, maybe I could run away from it. After most of a year, my final leg deposited me in the Caribbean, on St. Thomas in the US Virgin Islands. A couple months of blackout drinking later, I ended up co-owner of a rock 'n' roll nightclub, World Headquarters, on nearby St. John. Now buried in the substance-abuse lifestyle, I smoked four packs of cigarettes per day, drank beer and rum from the time I woke up until the time I passed out, and added as much speed, in its various guises, as my heart could handle without exploding. When a DEA agent investigating Caribbean cocaine distribution got stabbed in my club, I panicked (paranoid that I'd be wrongly implicated in the stabbing or cocaine trade) and fled back to mainland USA. And tried to turn things around. I got married, started running again, coached high school track, coached club cross country, returned to school, and thrilled to the birth of my son, Sean. And then, as was my modus operandi, I threw it all away to return to a life of drinking, smoking, and drugging. By age thirty-six, I was divorced, jobless, broke, and a few weeks away from homelessness (again). Desperate, I asked a friend in the film industry to send me some screenplays, so that I could see how they were done. I read the scripts, then banged out one of my own, *www.death.com*, and was signed by the agency CAA. That script didn't sell, but two months later my second one did, to New Line Cinema. And a month later, I signed to do a script rewrite for Disney. I moved into a nice house, began working more and sleeping less, and, naturally, increased my drinking and drugging. And a little over a year later, I ended up in the Verdugo Hills ER. Which is where you came in.

Film character Buckaroo Banzai famously said (OK, it's possible he pilfered it from Confucius or some other non-celluloid source), "No matter where you go, there you are." While I lack Banzai's multidimensional experience, I've always taken that to mean that you can't change your life or who you are by changing your location. On my travels across the country and around the world, I'd always been disappointed to discover that no matter how much geography I put between myself and my past behavior, I could never shake the person responsible for that behavior: me. And it was never long before I was repeating that behavior in my new location. And then fleeing to some other city or country or continent.

And attempts to target specific behaviors themselves—no matter my location—didn't work any better. I tried to quit smoking by throwing away my Marlboros. And to stop drinking by pouring bourbon down the drain. And to avoid the more extreme elements of my lifestyle by avoiding the people and places I associated with that behavior. But it never worked for long, because the problem wasn't cigarettes, liquor, drugs, people, or places.

The problem was me.

And the challenge was finding a way to change *me*.

Your challenge will be similar. Please don't take this the wrong way, but there's a reason that the change you're looking to make in your life is not already a part of your life. The obstacles that have prevented you from running in the past won't magically disappear the first time you don running shoes. In fact, the only way to overcome those obstacles will be to change the mentality of the person lacing up the shoes. You'll need to change yourself.

Lao-Tzu wrote, "A journey of a thousand miles begins with a single step."

That made sense to me. So on my thirty-ninth birthday, I stepped out the door for my first run in years. And I set a goal: Run fifteen minutes out, then fifteen minutes back.

That was a mistake. I made it five minutes. To the first traffic light. Then sat on the curb—gasping, trembling, and sweating—for another fifteen minutes. Then walked home. A friend of mine, Charlene, a fitness instructor, was there to greet me. "What'd you expect?" she said, shaking her head. "You're fat, you're middle-aged, and you smoke."

She was right. What had I expected? I hadn't treated the run like my first step in a "journey of a thousand miles." Instead, I'd ambushed my body. I'd tried to shock it into submission, the same way I tried to coax out extra pages of writing by tossing back whiskey shots.

The next day, I changed my approach. I visualized my end goal—running comfortably again—and then imagined all the workouts it would take to realize that outcome. And instead of putting myself through another self-inflicted five-minute body slam, I alternated walking and easy jogging for fifteen minutes. And then the next day, I began incrementally building from there. It was five months before I ran five miles continuously. And another year before I toed the line for my first race as a masters (age forty and over) runner.

I never again experienced the drop-dead fatigue that had derailed my first run, even as my long run edged up to fourteen miles and I added all manner of "speed work" (e.g., intervals, hill runs, hill repeats, sprints, drills, etc.) to my fitness routine. Running evolved from a chore into an eagerly anticipated break from the daily grind. My workouts became a time to unwind. A time to let my mind run free. And a time each day when I could experience the exhilaration that accompanies physical exertion, when I could marvel at the renewed strength, coordination, flexibility, and endurance that training had made possible. While I was running, I felt young again. And fit again. And vital. Believe it or not, I was having fun.

But the most amazing transformation in my life wasn't the improvement in my running. A few weeks into my training, I began cutting back on cigarettes before my run. Then I cut back after the run, too. And then I quit altogether. Evening runs began to take the place of evening drinks, which led to better sleep and the disappearance of morning jitters. When my screenplays with New Line and Disney went into turnaround (a death knell for most scripts), I didn't reach for a whiskey. I shrugged my shoulders—because the truth was that I wasn't much of a screenwriter, anyway; I'd been lucky with those sales, and no late-night writing meant no late-night amphetamines. I found a job that paid the rent, allowed me time to run, and freed up enough of every day to be a good father.

It turned out that I was also a pretty good runner for my age. Over the next decade, I'd win six individual masters national cross country titles, lead my masters club to nineteen team national championships in cross country and road racing, and set multiple American age-group records, including fastest-ever times for age fifty-plus at 5K (15:01) and 10K (31:11), as well as the second-fastest time ever for the half marathon (1:10:19). I became a senior writer and columnist for *Running Times* magazine, and a contributor to *Runner's World* and *Competitor*.

Over the past fifteen years, since that first aborted run on my thirty-ninth birthday, I've probably logged in the neighborhood of forty thousand miles. But my journey has carried me much further than that. Frankly, I feel like I've been to the moon and back.

This book is called *The Born Again Runner* because I truly believe that a successful running program can change your life. It can help you achieve your fitness goals, certainly, but it can also provide a blueprint for living the rest of your life: It can show you how putting your faith in small, incremental, present-day changes can lead to transformational outcomes in the future. If you're like me, it will give you the confidence to adopt a similar approach toward other aspects of your life, whether that means weight loss, career aspirations, improved interpersonal relationships, overcoming addiction and other health issues, or dealing with any other obstacle that stands between you and your goals.

On the other hand, if all you're looking for is a running program—if you're not signing on for a life makeover—don't worry, because running is what this book is about. It will guide you from your first step out the door through the successful implementation of your running program. You'll be provided with a step-by-step plan for improving your fitness that includes sample training programs, injury-prevention exercises, and an entire chapter devoted to creating your personal action plan.

But even before you begin training, *The Born Again Runner* will prepare you, mentally and practically, for your new program. You'll learn how to overcome excuses, body-related misconceptions, and health issues that have held you back in the past. You'll be introduced to twelve "guiding principles" that, once embraced, will ensure a successful start to your program. You'll get advice on proper attire. Learn the "rules of the road," regardless of where you train: your neighborhood, parks, trails, the local high school track—anywhere your feet can carry you. You'll be forewarned about common training errors. And you'll be advised on how to utilize the multifaceted running community as a support group for the journey ahead.

Finally, this book includes one runner profile per chapter. These are stories of runners who made the decision to start or restart a running program. You'll read about their motivations, the obstacles they faced, and the successes they achieved. Some of you will see your own issues in these profiles. All of you, I think, will relate to the runners' struggles.

When I wrote my first running book, *Build Your Running Body*, with coauthors Melissa Breyer and Tom Schwartz, I focused almost entirely on the physiological principles of training. I broke the body into its various components (e.g., muscles, connective tissue, cardiovascular system, nervous system, etc.), and I explained exactly how each component worked and how to train it. The finished book succeeded in conveying the most up-to-date information on every aspect of training, nutrition, competition, and full-body strengthening. And part of me figured I'd said all I had to say on the topic of running.

But after conversations with my editor at The Experiment and with a few close friends, I began to believe that there might be a second running book in me. Because while *Build Your Running Body* had created a science-driven manual for the sport, it hadn't really touched upon the visceral and often tentative first steps we must take to join the sport. It hadn't documented the long and winding road I'd traveled—that we must *all* travel—during our running journeys. In short, I hadn't fully explored the "two sides of Pete," as my editor put it. My first book had tapped the side represented by the record-holding masters runner and coach, but it was the other side—the self-destructive and monumentally imperfect man who'd donned running shoes simply to survive—who needed to speak.

The Born Again Runner is that second book.

Back in 2000, an ER physician told me that I might not live to see my son graduate from high school. On a warm June evening in 2012, I sat in the South Pasadena High School stands—fit, healthy, and thinking back on a decade-plus of wonderful times spent with my son—and watched Sean get his diploma. That was easily the greatest accomplishment of my life.

Now it's your turn.

Pete Magill

January 29, 2016

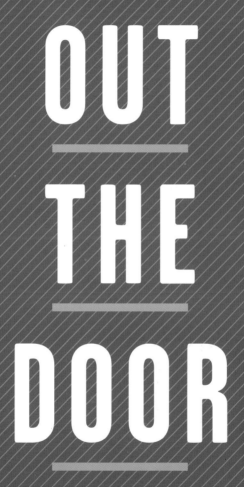

PART ONE

OUT THE DOOR

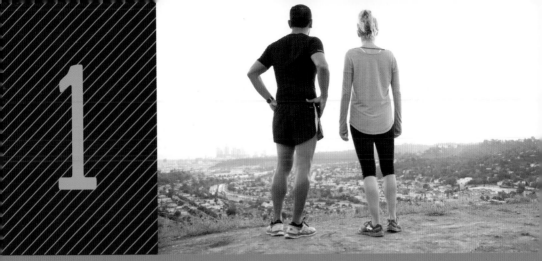

Give Me Your Tired, Your Overweight,

Your Out-of-Shape, Your First-Time, Your Addicted, Your Old, Your Injured, Your People with Disabilities, Your Reluctant Runners Yearning to Breathe Freely

"Everyone is an athlete. The only difference is that some of us are in training, and some are not."

—DR. GEORGE SHEEHAN

WAS TWENTY-FOUR YEARS OLD the first time a doctor told me I should never run again. It was a Monday, two days after a Southern California road race, and my lower back muscles were as tight as a soldier's newly made bed—you could bounce a quarter off them.

"Hmm," said the doctor, studying an X-ray of my spine, "this isn't good."

I could see the X-ray, too. But given that it would be a decade before I took an anatomy class at Glendale College or volunteered in the trauma center at USC County General, I had no idea what horror he'd spotted.

"Right here," he said, and pointed toward the curve of my lumbar vertebrae, just above my tailbone. "Those vertebrae aren't lined up correctly. When you run, the impact causes them to slide even further out of line. Frankly, you're lucky you're just having back spasms. If those vertebrae slip enough to damage your spinal cord, well, you won't have to worry about running again—you might never *walk* again."

The next day, I informed my coach that I was never going to run again.

And then, the following Saturday, with my back spasms having subsided, I changed my mind and ran another race. I finished well. So I decided to keep training for a little while longer. I've probably logged about fifty thousand miles in the years since.

And, yes, my spine is fine. Thank you for asking.

You see, I was suffering from lower back spasms (see page 252 for an exercise, the daydreamer, to alleviate these spasms in five to ten minutes). Not a deformed skeleton.

The point isn't that runners shouldn't listen to doctors. We should and do, although a second (and sometimes third and fourth) opinion should be part of that process.

The point is that just because someone says you can't run doesn't mean you can't run. *Especially if that someone is yourself.* After all, if a doctor can make a mistake about your ability to run, so can you.

BECOMING A BORN AGAIN RUNNER

If you're reading this book, I'm going to assume that you want to run. Or are thinking about running. Or know someone whom you feel should consider running.

And I'm also going to assume, since you're reading this book, that there's some obstacle, great or small, preventing you from launching full-bore into your running program. It might be a physical impediment. It might be some preconceived notion of what's required to run. It might be a motivational issue. Or it could be as rudimentary as not knowing where to start.

So the very first thing I want to tell you is this: *Relax. Take a deep breath. Exhale.*

If you want to run, you can run.

It's as simple as that.

It will require patience, planning, and a willingness to commit to a sensible and effective program. But assuming that sounds agreeable, this book will provide all the information you need in order to achieve your personal running goals.

And before some of you roll your eyes and assume that this is yet another exercise book that overestimates your fitness level and underestimates the challenges you face, I promise you that this book takes nothing for granted. Even in the best of circumstances, it's not easy to transition from non-runner to runner. Add in factors like weight, age, stress, career, and family obligations—not to mention more serious health issues like heart disease, osteoporosis, addiction, and limb amputation—and the act of lacing up running shoes can take on the intimidating aura of a steep glacier ascent to the summit of Mount Everest.

But again, relax. We're going to take this slowly. And, as your guide for this journey, I assure you that I've navigated the path before. If this *was* Everest, I'd be your Sherpa. I know the route. And I know the dangers. And by the time we've finished our journey, you'll know them, too.

If you've read this book's Introduction (and I recommend that you do), then you know that my own running journey included a long struggle with substance abuse. And you also know that, although I've enjoyed successes as both an athlete and a coach, my primary running accomplishment was reclaiming control of my life.

If this book has a mission, it's to offer you the same opportunity: the chance to use running as a medium for change, to affect your own life in a positive manner. You get to determine the nature of that change. Maybe you just want to run a mile comfortably. Maybe you want to race a marathon. Maybe running is only a tool for effecting some other change—for losing weight or reducing stress or getting your primary care physician off your back during your yearly physical. Or maybe, like it was for me, running is the first step in a complete life makeover. Whatever change you're after, this book will do its best to help you get there.

But before we can do that, before we can start down the path to running fitness, you'll have to take the first step by yourself.

Your first step won't be a physical one. (Cue the applause from those who are relieved that it's not yet time to abandon the safe haven of the couch.) Instead, the first step takes place in the six to seven inches between your ears.

And it goes like this: *I will run.*

Not *I might.* Not *If only I could.* Not *Someday....*

But, "I will run."

You have to know you're going to run.

Because when you *know* you're going to run, it creates a fundamental shift in the way you approach training. When you truly accept that no excuse or rationalization is going to keep you from lacing up your running shoes and stepping out the door (workout after workout until you achieve your running goals), you become willing to do all the seemingly small and inconvenient things that it takes to sustain a running program—things like injury-prevention exercises, maintaining a healthy diet, and scheduling proper recovery post-exercise. In other words, knowing you're going to succeed and doing what's necessary to accomplish that success are *not* two separate things; they're flip sides of the same coin.

LEARNING TO LAUGH AT OURSELVES

"I joined the local health club on a special—$29 a month. But I haven't lost a pound. Apparently, you have to show up?" —Unknown

"RUNNING" ISN'T ALWAYS RUNNING

Of course, now that I've demanded that you declare your intention to run, it's time to take a step backward and acknowledge that a running program isn't always about "running." Especially in the beginning. Some of us aren't ready to run right out of the gate. "Walk before you run" may be a cliché, but it also happens to be good advice.

There is no generic, one-size-fits-all approach to beginning your running program. There is no requirement to run a certain distance. No universal prescription to maintain a certain effort level or pace. In fact, there is no reason you need to start by running at all. You can walk. Or do some resistance training. Or prep your body with some cross training. Or try a mix of all three. And, of course, if you *are* ready to run, you can do that, too.

To begin a running program, all you're obligated to do is rise from the couch, walk to the door, cross the threshold, and be prepared to do *something*.

And the only unbreakable rule for your first workout is this: It shouldn't leave you so exhausted or disenchanted that you don't want to do a second workout.

Sound reasonable?

You'd be surprised.

A few years ago, my neighbor from down the street, Alan, stopped by to discuss his first day of running after a four-month break for a foot injury. "Last week, I finally decided to test the foot," said Alan. "So I ran six miles. The next day, my foot was hurting all over again. So I guess that's that." Actually, what's what is that Alan self-sabotaged his return to running by exercising too hard, too soon. His untrained body wasn't ready for six miles—*regardless of what he might have been running four months earlier*—and his foot broke down. (If it hadn't been his foot, it would have been something else, a knee or a hip or his shins.) This wasn't bad luck. It was inevitable.

Unfortunately, some runners think that a hard first day is an essential element of a serious training program. They think it shows commitment. Or jump-starts their fitness. Or some other nonsense. So they blast off the start line for that first run as if some race official had just fired a pistol. And then, a few minutes later, red-faced, chest heaving, legs aching, they collapse in a puddle of fatigue. The next day, they're back on the couch, their bodies paralyzed by severe muscle soreness (a condition known as "delayed-onset muscle soreness," better known by its acronym, DOMS), wondering why on earth anyone would make a habit out of running.

The good news is that you don't have to make this mistake.

Running hard at the outset of a running program assumes two things: first, that your body already knows how to run; and second, that your body is ready for a challenging effort. As you'll discover in the coming chapters, neither assumption is correct. The act of running is a learned skill, not an innate one, and endurance is earned through weeks and months of training, not through birthright. As such, you'll be launching your program with very manageable workouts. In fact, your first few weeks of training just might be, dare I say, *pleasant*.

BORN TO WALK AND JOG (SLOWLY)

The topic of innate running ability deserves another moment of our attention. Mostly because some of you might be familiar with a theory that suggests you were, in fact, "born to run." And because you might be worried that, if the theory is true, evolution has somehow passed you by—you know, since jogging to the corner and back leaves you sucking wind and drenched in sweat.

Don't worry. There's nothing wrong with you. *No one* is ready to run on the first day.

It's become fashionable in the twenty-first century to seek a return to our roots. I don't mean our hometowns or our parents' hometowns or our grandparents' or great-grandparents' places of origin. I refer to the roots of our evolutionary forebears—you know, the *cavemen*.

Faced with a complex modern world, it's comforting to retreat into what evolutionary biologist and author Marlene Zuk has dubbed *paleo-fantasy*, a pseudoscientific belief that human physiology has remained the same since the time of cavemen and that mimicking the caveman's (mythical) lifestyle will leave us healthier, fitter, and happier.

With this in mind, some dieters eat a paleo diet.

And some runners have embraced a theory that proclaims humans to be the beneficiaries of an evolution-delivered endurance inheritance. For these runners, the theory goes like this: *Australopithecus*, our pre-*Homo* ancestor, climbed down from the trees four million years ago and began hunting the tasty, four-legged morsels populating the African savanna. Roughly two million years later, this hunting paid off with evolutionary adaptations in *Homo habilis* and *Homo erectus* that included improvements in tendons, arches, butt, balance, stride length, and sweat glands. The upshot was that our ancestors could now run long distances in pursuit of high-calorie prey (an activity known as a "persistence hunt"), and this running ability subsequently became a driver of human evolution (just as the high-calorie prey became the evolutionary antecedent to modern barbecue).

Therefore, in theory, we're all genetically predisposed—or "born"—to run distance.

But there's a problem with this theory.

For starters, if we modern humans are the evolutionary spawn of distance runners, born into the world with virtual Boston Marathon competitors' bibs safety-pinned to our chests, how do we explain a 50 percent annual injury rate for runners (shod or shoeless—and don't worry, you'll learn in this book how to be part of the 50 percent who remain healthy), the fact that only 16 percent of Americans willingly engage in daily exercise (as opposed to 95 percent who watch TV every day), or, let's get real, the very existence of the Dallas Cowboys' offensive line? If we're born preprogrammed for endurance activity, we have a funny way of showing it. And science simply doesn't support the claim. A 2015 article in the *Quarterly Review of Biology* credits the consumption of plant foods, which contain high concentrations of carbohydrates (in contrast to the protein derived from hunts), with driving evolution of "the brain and other human traits." As for the persistence hunts themselves, most researchers believe that the "running" in those hunts was, in reality, restricted to long periods of walking combined with surges of slow jogging. So, at best, this is what you were "born" to do: walk and maybe jog occasionally.

Followed by some carbs for your post-walking-and-jogging snack.

And that's a more realistic start line for most runners—not to mention a relief to those of you who have never felt the urge to launch into a spontaneous twelve-hour footrace with area wildlife or your neighbor's dog.

Don't get me wrong. You *do* possess the potential to become a runner. Just as you possess the potential to dribble a basketball, become a pastry chef, or graduate from college. It's just that you don't get that for free. No legacy running here. You have to earn it.

RUNNING HAS SOMETHING FOR EVERY BODY

Of course, you don't need science to tell you that we aren't the evolutionary offspring of a single race of inexhaustible distance runners.

All you have to do is take a look around you.

We humans come in all shapes and sizes, and, more to the point of this book, runners come in all shapes and sizes.

Sure, the winner of the Olympic Marathon (or Boston or London or pretty much any major marathon worldwide) is going to sport a different body type than the donut-inhaling security guard at the mall. But that doesn't mean that only humans with the same body type as marathon champions have the potential to become runners, any more than a donut-inhaling security guard has sole dibs on the apple fritters at your local Dunkin' Donuts.

The concept of body types was hatched by American psychologist William Sheldon, back in the 1940s, as a way to (arbitrarily) categorize people based upon their shape:

→ **Ectomorph:** A lean machine with long thin limbs, flat chest, equal shoulder and hip width, and low body fat. Ectomorphs seem incapable of gaining weight but have an equally hard time putting on muscle.

→ **Mesomorph:** A muscular Greek god(dess) with wide shoulders and powerful chest, narrow waist, hips about equal width as the shoulders, and great definition from head to toe. Strong and speedy, destined to be the top jocks in high school.

→ **Endomorph:** Soft and curvy, a tendency toward a pear shape, with fat tending to follow gravity and settle in the lower body. Voluptuous females, and males who sport that spare tire around the waist.

There's only one problem with these three categories: The vast majority of real-life people don't fit into any of them. We're a combination of all three—and then some.

Yes, most marathon champions could double as the photo illustration for an encyclopedia entry on "ectomorph." And yes, these ectomorphic champions do seem to scoot freely down the road like leaves driven before a blustery wind.

But no, that doesn't mean that only ectomorphs can become runners.

Seriously, if that isn't you, so what? That isn't me, either, and I've logged tens of thousands of miles. That isn't 90 percent of the fifty million Americans who go for a jog every year or the fifteen million who completed a race in 2015. (Don't believe me? Just head down to a local 5K and watch runners crossing the finish line.)

Percentage of Total Body Types

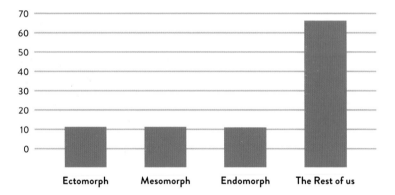

No body type comes ready-built for running. That's because running adaptations have nothing to do with body type. Most are invisible to the naked eye. They involve your heart, your blood vessels, your bones, your muscle cells, your nervous system, and your mind.

So when you look into the mirror and fail to see your running potential, it isn't because there's no potential there. It's because you're failing to see the actual person staring back at you.

It's a uniquely human trait to find patterns where there are none. We see a man in the moon. Animals in clouds. Or the Virgin Mary on a slice of burnt toast. And many of us, when we look into the mirror, see something other than our real bodies. We see a pattern—an extrapolation of a lifetime's worth of negative associations with our body type. We see years of negative messaging from the media, convincing us of our inability to measure up to the "ideal" body images depicted via TV, the Internet, magazines, billboards, and video games. We project the "constructive criticism" of well-meaning family members and friends. And we incorporate the spiteful asides of acquaintances and strangers.

We accept this false image of ourselves and act as if the limitations associated with that image are, in fact, real. But they're not.

You are not a body type.

And you are not a stone, incapable of transformation. You are a living, breathing person on the brink of reimagining your life and re-creating your image.

And so when you look into the mirror, this is what I want you to see: a runner.

Because there is no mold from which we runners are cast. There is no Rorschach inkblot test to illuminate our suitability for the sport. And there is no preexisting condition—especially body type—that disqualifies us from lacing up our shoes and heading out the door.

REALITY LEAVES A LOT TO THE IMAGINATION

So what's standing between you and your first step out the door?

It's not fitness; there is no workout so small that it can't launch your running program. And it's not evolution; running is learned, not innate. And it's not body type; any correlation between body shape and your ability to benefit from an exercise routine is an illusion.

Still, there's something that's been holding you back.

And I understand that your *something* is very real to you.

But reality is malleable.

Copernicus proved that the earth revolves around the sun. Darwin rewrote the history of all life with his theory of evolution. Einstein shattered our notion of time by illustrating that it stops for objects traveling the speed of light.

If there is one thing we can say about "reality," it's that it's seldom up to speed with the complex nature of our world—or of our potential to act within it.

It's the same with your reality. In the chapters ahead, we'll address the specific obstacles to running (e.g., weight, age, biomechanics, medical issues, environment, etc.) that you fear are too large to overcome. And we'll explain in detail how to incorporate an effective running program into any lifestyle. And, of course, we'll work together to create the best possible running schedule for achieving your personal goals.

BECOMING A RUNNER: *Mike Hutchins*

Mike Hutchins, of Grand Prairie, Texas, now age fifty-four, was in his midforties when he began to experience severe pain in his legs and glutes (butt) while walking. "I couldn't go a hundred yards before I'd have to take a break," says Mike. "I'd be mowing the yard and have to quit after a couple strips." Referred to a cardiologist, Mike was diagnosed with peripheral artery disease (PAD) and partially blocked carotid arteries—his doctor said Mike had the arteries of an eighty-year-old. In PAD, the capillaries (small blood vessels) that bring oxygen to muscles begin to shrink and disappear, leading to the death of muscle cells themselves. Mike underwent surgery, receiving stents for his aorta and iliac arteries. The improvement in his walking was immediately apparent, and Mike decided he wanted to try running—an activity he'd last attempted as a freshman in high school, when he'd run hurdles. "I just decided to run a 5K," says Mike, and he set himself a goal of sub-30 minutes. So at age forty-eight, Mike went for his first run in decades. He lasted one minute. "And I felt like I was going to die," he says. But Mike had made a commitment, so he ran again, and at four weeks experienced a sharp pain between his shoulders. An X-ray was inconclusive, but the pain stopped Mike from running for six

For now, I'm going to ask you to have faith that the answers to your running questions will be answered. And I'm also going to ask you to finish what we started earlier in this chapter.

It's time for you to take your first step.

It's time for you to say out loud, "I will run."

Or if you're an introvert uncomfortable with audible declarations, it's time to promise yourself, visualizing each word as you do: *I will run.*

And that's all it takes. With that simple declaration, you're on your way to becoming a *born again runner.* This is not a religious definition. And

months. Refusing to give up, he tried again—and felt another sharp pain in his back. This time, an MRI revealed three compression fractures in his spine. A subsequent bone-density scan led to a diagnosis of idiopathic osteoporosis. Mike was prescribed Forteo, a bone-building drug he'd have to inject for two years. "That's as long as you can use it," he says. "Something about cancer in mice and all that stuff." One year later, he was back in his running shoes, and soon after that he walked/ran his first 5K in 37:32. Three years later, after three 10Ks, one 15K, three half marathons, one marathon, and fifty-seven 5Ks, Mike finally accomplished his goal of a sub-30-minute 5K, running 29:41 at the St. Maria Goretti 5K, in Arlington, Texas, on May 9, 2015. Asked about the most important aspect of his training, Mike doesn't hesitate. "Patience," he says. "Don't believe everything you read—don't believe *anything* you read. That's for normal people. If it says it takes six weeks, it takes me six months." For those who suffer from PAD, he offers this encouragement: "Do what you can—but *do!*"

it's not a miraculous conversion of your soul (we'll save that for your first "runner's high"—the sense of Zen-like euphoria that fit runners often experience during their training outings). Instead, it is a statement of action.

For the remainder of this book, we won't use the terms "new runner" or "returning runner" unless specifically identifying information pertinent to each group (e.g., injury-prevention advice for returning runners who've suffered chronic injuries in the past).

From now on, you're a runner. Period.

CHAPTER TAKEAWAY

If you want to run, you can run. Running doesn't discriminate—it's not based on genetics, body type, or whatever personal obstacles you face. Of course, success in a running program demands patience and planning. But beginning that running program doesn't demand anything more than commitment to see your program through, internalized by your declaration: "I will run." Beginning a running program doesn't even demand that you run; instead, it simply requires that you initiate some exercise that will carry you closer to your long-term running goal. It asks you to reimagine your life as the end-product of those running goals and to have faith in yourself and your program to turn that imagined life into reality.

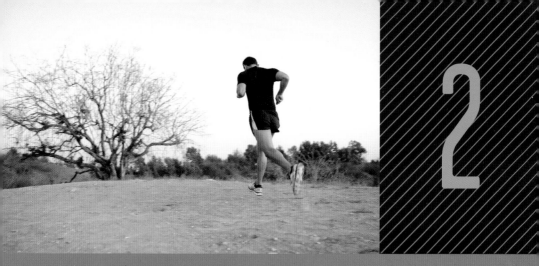

Twelve Guiding Principles for a Born Again Runner

"If you don't have time to do it right,
when will you have time to do it over?"
—JOHN WOODEN

THERE'S AN OLD JOKE ABOUT CIGARETTES: "It's easy to quit smoking. I've done it a hundred times."

I used to be a smoker, so the joke resonates with me. I quit when I was seventeen. And then at nineteen. And twenty. And twenty-one. And twenty-seven. And thirty-two. And finally, once and for all, at age thirty-nine. And then again at age forty-one (so shoot me, I fell off the wagon for a few weeks). I've been holding steady ever since.

The same pattern holds true for my experience with starting a running program. I've done it a dozen (OK, a few dozen) times, often in tandem with a vow to quit smoking. Most of these start-ups involved an inflated sense of my day one readiness. Then a sinking feeling during my kickoff run when my legs, arms, and shoulders turned to stone, and then to liquid fire, often followed by dizziness and a quick decision to *Abort! Abort!* And then, the next day, the same thing all over again. And then a few more days like that. Until finally I'd have to concede that I wasn't ready for the new program, after which I'd stow the running shoes and promise myself that I'd try again in the future. When I was better prepared. When I'd lost some weight, or quit smoking, or my horoscope gave me a thumbs-up, or you fill in the blank.

It's good to have a sense of humor about botched attempts to get fit. It doesn't erase the pain of overzealous first runs or the sense of failure when our programs crumble. But it does allow us to make peace with the fact that we are human. And it sets the stage for exhibiting one of our most indispensable human attributes: our resilience—our willingness to *try, try again.*

But resilience by itself won't ensure success with a new running program. Not if your program is simply a repeat of previous mistakes. Instead, you'll need a game plan. In Part II of this book, you'll learn how to build a smart, effective, and personalized training schedule. But that's not the "game plan" I'm talking about. Your game plan is bigger than your schedule. It's the overarching philosophy that will guide all your decisions as a runner—from molding your self-image to planning your diet to, yes, of course, choosing your workouts.

Many of the principles that you'll integrate into your game plan will be drawn from your unique experiences, but some principles are universal and best embraced at the outset of your program. The following twelve are a good place to start.

PRINCIPLE 1: THE PAST IS THE PAST

If you attempted to start a running program in the past and failed, so what? Get over it. There's nothing shameful or even original about failure. We all fail in our attempts at running (or at anything else in life) until we do this: We succeed.

As a sophomore, Michael Jordan failed to make his high school's varsity basketball team, even as his friend and fellow sophomore Leroy

Smith did, inspiring Jordan to work harder than ever, an attitude that eventually carried him to six NBA titles and recognition as one of the greatest basketball players of all time. Jordan's story is hardly unique. Steven Spielberg was rejected by the renowned USC film school before going on to become the highest-grossing director of all time, with box office grosses exceeding nine billion dollars. The Beatles flunked their 1962 audition with Decca Records, who opined that the band had "no future in show business." And Dr. Seuss had his first children's book rejected by twenty-seven publishers.

What, you didn't live up to a New Year's Eve resolution? Maybe you started a running program and didn't finish it? Or planned a program and never even started it? Congratulations, that makes you exactly like 70 to 80 percent of all people who set fitness goals.

Or maybe it's more serious than a failed New Year's resolution. Maybe there's a medical condition, a struggle with addiction, or other significant issue that's kept you from lacing up your running shoes. It's natural to feel hesitant in those situations. *Hesitant.* Not immobilized. Not terrified. As Nobel Prize–winning author William Faulkner wrote, "You cannot swim for new horizons until you have courage to lose sight of the shore."

The opportunity to succeed exists only when you try.

LEARNING TO LAUGH AT OURSELVES

"My coach said that the most important parts of running are loosening up first and stretching out after. So I drank six beers and took a nap." —Unknown

PRINCIPLE 2: WALK BEFORE YOU RUN

Yes, it's a cliché (as noted in Chapter 1). But it's also true.

Walk before you jog. Jog before you run. Run easy before you run harder.

There's a reason why you can't launch your running program with hard workouts beginning on day one. It's because your body isn't ready. Your muscles aren't strong enough. Your fuel supplies aren't large enough. Your blood can't carry enough oxygen. Your nervous system has no idea how to properly control your legs or torso or arms while running; in effect, you're a puppet with tangled strings. Train too hard on a body that's not ready, and it's like driving your car across a papier-mâché bridge—the bridge is going to collapse.

There's a term in fitness called *specificity of training*. I know, that sounds complicated, but it's actually a simple concept: You improve at specific types of exercise by performing that exercise. This means that if you haven't been running (or, at least, performing exercises to strengthen your body in anticipation of running), your body isn't prepared to run. Take your muscles. When you start a running program, exercise damages your out-of-shape muscle cells. The harder you exercise, the more damage you inflict. That's because harder efforts use more muscle cells (e.g., you use fewer muscle cells to jog than to sprint, and fewer still to walk than to jog). Unfortunately, your body can only repair a small amount of muscle damage each day. If you train too hard, your body can't keep up with the repairs. Your muscles ache, and your body winds up back on the couch. Better to start with an easy effort, such as walking. Once your body has repaired and fortified the muscle cells used for that activity, you can increase your intensity—say, to jogging. Then repair. Then train a little harder. And repair again. And keep going until you've reached your goal distance and effort.

If you train too much, too soon, you won't get fit. You'll get sore.

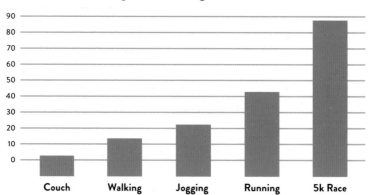

Percentage of Running Muscle Cells Used

PRINCIPLE 3: KEEP IT SIMPLE

Don't overorchestrate your initial workouts.

To echo Nike's advertising slogan: *Just run.* Or just walk. Or just do some resistance training. Or some easy cross training.

The success of your running program will be determined by action, not grand gestures. You don't need to pick a special launch day, such as New Year's, your birthday, or National Running Day (which, by the way, is the first Wednesday in June). You don't need a scenic route. Or a sunrise. Or a sunset. Or the theme from *Rocky*.

You need a run, period.

It's best to pick a practical route, one that is free from obstacles and doesn't carry you far from your start line. A local track is perfect. Or a residential block. Or a short loop in the park. And the best time to schedule your run is (drumroll, please): today.

PRINCIPLE 4: SHIRT, SHORTS, SHOES

Don't over-shop your initial training gear.

All you need to begin your program is a running shirt, a pair of running shorts, and a pair of running shoes. If you want to go nuts: two shirts, two pairs of shorts, and two pairs of shoes.

A few years ago, my friend Sam asked me to create a training schedule for him. He was super excited after spending the day shopping for new gear. He'd bought training and racing shoes, a half dozen matched outfits (shirts and shorts), a Gore-Tex warm-up suit, and a GPS watch with a heart-rate monitor. "I'm ready to go!" he said. When I asked if he'd gone for a run yet, he said, "I needed to motivate myself first." Which explained the day's purchases. After a few days, I had Sam's schedule ready for him. But I couldn't find Sam. He didn't call me. He didn't drop by my house. When I eventually ran into Sam several weeks later, he admitted he'd lost interest in running—without having attempted so much as a jog around the block.

Sam had expended his enthusiasm on shopping. There was none left for actual running.

Run first. Then buy gear and gadgets as your training requires.

It's a mental thing. You're either starting your running program, or you're delaying it.

PRINCIPLE 5: TRAIN WITH THE BODY YOU HAVE

Runners come in all shapes and sizes, and they hail from every fitness (or lack-of-fitness) background imaginable. But you don't. You come in only one model: you.

We discussed "body type" in Chapter 1. But we're talking about more than body type here. We're talking about your unique physical characteristics. About your gender. Your age. Your weight. Your fitness background. Your heart rate. Your nervous system efficiency. Your ratio of endurance-oriented muscle cells (slow-twitch) to sprinter-type muscle cells (fast-twitch). Your stride mechanics. Your capacity to produce aerobic energy—or to weather the fatigue-inducing by-products of anaerobic energy production. And much more.

Every runner is different. If we were plotting our fitness journeys on a map, we'd need separate pushpins because each of us would be starting from a different location. Each of us would require a slightly different route on our journey to the distant land of "fit runner." When you attempt to emulate the training of some other runner (of a friend or an acquaintance or even some elite runner whom you admire) or to follow generic workout schedules found in magazines and books (the reason this book offers multiple workout options), remember that those programs have a different start point than yours. It's like trying to drive from Los Angeles to New York City using directions cribbed from someone who began his or her journey in Miami.

Your body won't magically adapt to any running program you choose. Instead, you have to choose a program that's suited to your unique body. And you must be willing to make adjustments to that program based upon feedback from your body.

PRINCIPLE 6: IT'S THE RECOVERY, STUPID!

Runners are sometimes surprised to learn that they don't get fit while exercising. They get fit while recovering from exercise.

This is what happens to you when you train: You apply enough physical stress to muscles, bones, and other tissues to cause minor damage (and trigger other rebuilding mechanisms), and you deplete your body's reserves of carbohydrate fuel, hormones, and other exercise-related substances.

This is what happens while you're recovering: Your body repairs the damage and restocks your depleted fuel and other substances—*and*, because your body wants to protect you against a similar fate in the future, it overcompensates during this phase, building stronger muscles, stronger bones, and a larger fuel supply, as well as instigating other adaptations that will make you a better runner in the future.

But this recovery process takes time—up to a day after easy outings, and between forty-eight and seventy-two hours following harder workouts. If you try to run hard every day, you interrupt this recovery process. Your body doesn't get the repairs it needs, and you break down.

This is why experienced runners employ a "hard-easy" approach to training. With hard-easy, you push yourself one day (although not to exhaustion), then take it easy the next. And as your running program becomes more demanding, you schedule an entire easy week every month, during which you lower your running volume and intensity—usually by shortening distance runs and scheduling fewer repetitions on interval days.

Bottom line: It's not the training you do that counts; it's the training from which you can recover.

PRINCIPLE 7: THE ONLY OPINION THAT MATTERS IS YOUR OWN

People are going to comment on your running program, and it won't all be compliments and high fives. Ignore the haters. Ignore the Negative Neds and Nellies.

My friend Scott Douglas, a senior content editor for *Runner's World* and coauthor of *Meb for Mortals*, wrote an essay, "The Fit Life: Running for Freedom," in which he recounts running past a convenience store every day. And every day, the same kids would loiter outside the store.

The kids would shout at Scott, "Hut, two, three, four . . . hut, two, three, four. . . ." Scott didn't take offense. Instead, he pitied the kids. "After all," he wrote, "running has made me freer than I ever could have imagined. . . . Rather than being yet another task on the day's to-do list, the run [is] a release, a time to explore, as far as possible from the regimentation implied by 'Hut, two, three, four.'" For Scott, running was freedom. And the kids' taunts were the antithesis of freedom, a reflexive need to mesh with the herd, to deride any action that lay outside the herd's experience.

As another example, more than thirty years ago my girlfriend at the time, Cathy, who was significantly overweight, launched her running program with a short jog on the road adjacent to Pasadena's Rose Bowl. A motorist pulled alongside her, rolled down his window, and yelled, "Give it up! It's too late for you!" Then he laughed like hell. Cathy was in tears that night. But she didn't *give it up*. And three decades later, Cathy is fit and looks fantastic, and that jerk is undoubtedly still a jerk.

By starting a running program, you are exercising your power to become the person you want to be. Don't relinquish that power—not for a second—to the infrequent negative comment.

It's untrue that "sticks and stones may break my bones, but names will never hurt me." Name-calling can hurt. It can hurt a lot. If it didn't, bullies wouldn't do it.

But then, as with the occasional calf cramp, shake it off and keep running.

PRINCIPLE 8: NO RAIN CHECKS UNLESS IT'S RAINING

Only skip workouts on days when you have no choice except to skip your workout.

There will inevitably be days when you can't run—when injury, excessive fatigue, subzero weather, illness, important social obligations (e.g., weddings, not TV shows), or some other obstacle prevents you from getting out the door. On those days, by all means take a rain check.

And then there will be days when you simply don't *feel* like running. Maybe you've had a long day at work. Or your running partner calls in sick.

Or a triple-scoop brownie sundae calls out to you. On these days, well, there's really no polite way to say this: Get your butt out the door and run!

A running program only works when you're working it. The incremental gains you make through long-term training can suffer a meteoric crash and burn if you begin to miss workouts. There are some fitness gains that have a half-life of one week, which means you lose half of *all* those gains after a single week of non-training, even if they required months to accrue. And on the mental side, you create a slippery slope when you begin justifying not exercising just *because*. In contrast, it takes only token runs to maintain fitness gains. And there's also this: Once you're out the door, you just might discover that you're glad to be running.

This doesn't mean you have to be like three-time Olympian and 1970 Boston Marathon champion Ron Hill, who never missed a day of running for fifty years—yes, 18,263 days, during which he accumulated 134,531 miles. Once, after bunion surgery, Hill hopped a twenty-seven-minute mile with a crutch to keep his streak alive. Another time, he trained the day after breaking his collarbone in a car crash. You don't have to do that. But you *do* have to acknowledge that if Hill could hop a mile with a crutch, you can run after a long day at work (or even, if we're being honest, when it *is* raining).

PRINCIPLE 9: DIETING CAN WAIT (AND SO CAN EVERYTHING ELSE)

Rome wasn't built in a day. The new you will take time to construct, too.

You've already committed to one major change in your life. You've committed to becoming a runner. Your running program will require time, energy (both physical and mental), and adjustments to your non-running schedule. The last thing you need at this point is additional change and stress.

From the American Psychological Association: "[Replacing] unhealthy behaviors with healthy ones requires time . . . To improve your success, focus on one goal or change at a time. As new healthy behaviors become a habit, try to add another goal that works toward the overall change you're striving for."

BECOMING A RUNNER:
Cori Canada Shuford

Cori Canada Shuford, age thirty-two, of Conway, South Carolina, who stands 5 feet 2 inches tall and weighed 260 pounds in December 2010, was mired in depression following the death of her daughter, Isabella, and three miscarriages. "Eating was the only thing I could control that comforted me," says Cori. "I'd leave work, go through the McDonald's drive-through, and supersize everything. Then I'd eat it all before I got home. I'd put it in the trash can so that my husband couldn't see it, then make dinner like a normal person." For Cori, weight control has been a lifelong struggle. She recalls standing in line in fifth grade, discussing weight with the other girls. "I said I weighed 100 pounds," says Cori, "and the girls were shocked." Cori played a little softball in high school, but she wasn't very good at it. "I was a cheerleader, too," she says, before adding, "a fat one." After her three miscarriages, Cori and her husband, Lance, adopted their first child, Zachary. Then Cori got pregnant again, with Isabella, but went into labor at twenty weeks. When Isabella died only hours after birth, Zachary was the reason Cori kept going. Later, she and Lance adopted Sophia. When Sophia was six months old, Cori got pregnant again. "I told God that if I was having another baby to have it die in my arms, then take it right there." New daughter Emma made it. And Cori began the process of forgiving herself. "For the longest time," she says, "I'd blamed myself [for Isabella's death], because it was my body that had failed her." Cori made a

I realize that many of you are starting your running program for the express purpose of losing weight. But be patient. At its outset, your running program will increase your hunger, making dieting more difficult. Additionally, dieting restricts the fuel your muscles have available, creating greater fatigue during exercise. That makes dieting a lose-lose proposition when you're trying to get your running program off the ground.

The good news is that you'll find it easier to start a diet in a few weeks' time. Your runs will get progressively longer, burning more fat. And your

2011 New Year's Eve resolution to lose weight. She bought a treadmill and started walking, tagging a one-minute run onto the end of her workout. "It was awful," she says of the first run. "I hated it. And I hated myself. I wondered why I was torturing myself." She built up to two minutes. Then to alternating a quarter-mile walk with a quarter-mile run. And six months after starting, she ran three miles without a break. By June, she'd lost fifty pounds. And the following November, with an assist from new training partner Liz—a coworker who introduced Cori to speed work and other technical aspects of running—Cori shocked herself by clocking 29:03 in her first 5K ever. "After I got over almost passing out," says Cori, "I felt—I don't even have a word for it—amazing, exhilarated. I never thought this 260-pound fat girl could run that fast." These days, Cori is about 160 pounds and a size 8. "I'm a single digit, and that's a big deal!" she says. And she has four half marathons under her belt. "There are times you feel like you're on top of the world, and you don't want to stop," says Cori about her running. "And if we don't get that feeling today, tomorrow we put on our shoes and try to get it again."

muscles will learn to store more energy, making them less reliant on daily calorie refortification.

Remember to focus on long-term goals. Your goal isn't to lose weight this week. It's to lose weight as the result of a sustainable program—and then to continue using that program to keep the weight off.

PRINCIPLE 10: SLOWER IS FASTER

Getting in shape takes time. Think months, not weeks—certainly not days. And regardless of the countless get-fit-quick schemes that populate the Internet, magazines, and television infomercials, there aren't any shortcuts.

When it comes to your running program, it's wise to remember *The Tortoise and the Hare.* In the well-known fable, the hare mocks the slower tortoise until the latter suggests a race. In the race, the tortoise's steady and consistent progress eventually bests the hare's poorly planned sprints and stops. Sure, it's only a story, and sure (as countless children have complained for countless generations) the hare should have won the stupid race. But the story is also a remarkably accurate metaphor for running. Runners who plan long-term advance in their programs at a predictable rate and usually achieve their goals. Runners who push too hard too fast end up (take your pick) injured, sick, burned out, or back on the couch.

The moral of the story is: The fastest way to become a successful runner is to take your time. Slower gets you there faster. Faster seldom gets you there at all.

PRINCIPLE 11: IT'S GOTTA BE FUN

If you don't enjoy running, you'll quit running.

It's that simple.

It's gotta be fun.

If the essential ingredient for running success were ice cream, not exercise, this book would be unnecessary. No one needs their arm twisted to down a bowl of chocolate peppermint crunch or vanilla caramel fudge.

Wanna keep running? Then make it fun. And you can start with these five suggestions:

1 PICK THE RIGHT WORKOUT: Exercising until it hurts isn't fun. So pick a workout that's manageable. That doesn't mean your workouts can't be challenging. They can. But "challenging" and "painful" are not synonyms—and the latter is a program killer.

2 CREATE A SUPPORT TEAM: Let close friends and family know you've started a running program. Then accept their praise as you achieve your goals. Don't be Batman, doing great deeds while hiding behind a mask.

3 SCHEDULE REWARDS: All stick and no carrot makes you an unhappy runner. Reward yourself with healthy and tasty snacks post-run. And give yourself a hefty bonus—dinner out, a movie, or a weekend getaway—when you accomplish something big.

4 JOIN THE RUNNING COMMUNITY: Run with friends, training groups, or clubs. Participate in online forums at runnersworld.com, runningahead.com, or letsrun.com. Visit a site like competitor.com for the latest fitness news or sportsscientists.com for in-depth, up-to-date, scientific analysis of exercise.

5 MAKE VARIETY THE SPICE OF RUNNING LIFE: Schedule a variety of workouts, from distance to tempo to form drills to resistance training (all discussed in the chapters ahead). If you need a day or two off from running, cross train.

Your running program shouldn't be an obligation. It should be a highlight of your day.

PRINCIPLE 12: KNOW YOU'LL SUCCEED

Yes, we discussed this in Chapter 1. But it bears repeating: You won't succeed in your running program until you truly believe that you will succeed.

When you know you're going to succeed, you become willing to do the things necessary to ensure that success:

→ You train at the correct effort level for the correct amount of time.

→ You include injury-prevention exercises post-workout.

→ You schedule recovery days—*and stick to the prescribed recovery workload.*

→ You don't skip runs.

→ You eat a healthy diet that provides the energy and nutrition required by your program.

→ You plan long-term; you think of where you want to be, fitness-wise, in months, not weeks (or days).

→ You resist impulsive, mid-workout decisions (e.g., racing someone who has the audacity to pass you during a distance run) that are dictated by ego rather than your predetermined exercise plan and legitimate feedback from your body.

→ You make exercise a scheduled part of your daily calendar, rather than continuously scrambling to clear an hour or two for your workouts.

When you know you're going to succeed, you don't worry that it will take three months to achieve your goals. Or six months. Or a year. You become like the painter who sees his finished art long before daubing the first strokes to the canvas. You're Michelangelo, who used his chisel to free David from a block of Carrara marble. You're already a runner, applying workouts with a steady hand, incrementally transforming your body to match an image that already exists in your mind.

CHAPTER TAKEAWAY

To succeed in running, you'll need more than good intentions and a workout schedule. You'll need an overarching game plan, a set of principles that will guide the creation of your program and provide solutions when things go wrong. First, you'll need to put previous fitness start-up failures out of your mind, because we all fail at our programs until we do this: We succeed. Next, you'll have to embrace a long-term approach to your running program. This will include a commitment to incremental training increases, proper recovery post-workout, patience when it comes to incorporating other fitness goals (e.g., weight loss), a realistic appraisal of your own fitness (and what program will work for you), and a refusal to let criticism, flagging motivation, or any other obstacle undermine your program. And, of course, you must find a way to keep running fun—if you don't, you'll stop running.

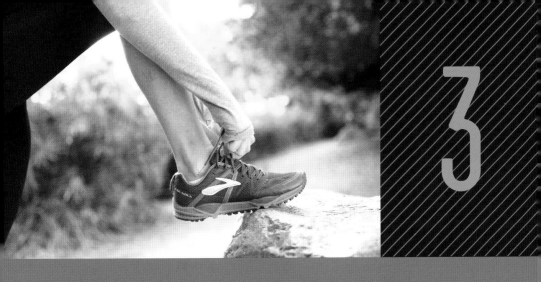

Myth Busting:
The No-Excuse Zone
(General)

"You can't wake a person who is
pretending to be asleep."
—NAVAJO PROVERB

SO ARE YOU READY TO RUN YET? I have a feeling that while some of you are ready to roll—have, in fact, been ready to charge out the door since your Chapter 1 declaration, "I will run!"— there are others who remain on the fence. And not because you're lazy. Not because you're afraid to commit. But because there are obstacles you face that don't simply vanish due to an adrenaline-fueled declaration of your intention to run. You want to run. Sure. But you aren't convinced that circumstances will *allow* you to run. Or that running will fit into your current lifestyle.

I get it. Honestly, there are so many reasons *not* to run that it's a miracle any of us laces up our running shoes. Potential runners don't have time, have no idea where to run, have no idea what to run, and are self-conscious about their weight, running form, training outfit, and rasping breath. Experienced runners are too tired, have that achy thing happening in their ankle, or can't because Bob or Betty or the rest of the gang can't make it today—and, really, who wants to run alone? Or there are the more serious (or serious-sounding) reasons: heart disease, osteoporosis, osteoarthritis, diabetes, drug addiction, menopause, and visual impairment. Or the fact that you recently blew out eighty or ninety candles on your birthday cake.

They're all good reasons. And I don't want you to think that I don't respect them.

But they're also this: excuses.

And as you'll soon discover, there are no "Get out of running free" cards in this book. With rare exceptions, everyone who *wants* to run *can* run. And every excuse that's holding you back is a hurdle somebody else has already cleared.

That said, I realize that these aren't just "excuses" to you. They're very real obstacles.

So for this chapter and the next, we're going to meet these issues head-on. Chapter 3 will focus on universal excuses that most runners entertain at one time or another. Chapter 4 will target biomechanical and medical excuses, as well as a few issues specific to female runners. Of course, covering every excuse in the book would require an entire (that's right) book, but we'll cover a lot of the biggies, and, in Chapter 4, we'll include interviews with experts on two major medical issues of concern to runners: heart disease and osteoporosis.

EXCUSE CATEGORY ONE: THE *TOOS*

If there is one category of excuses to which no potential runner is immune, it's the *toos*. We're simply *too something-or-other* to start a running program. Too heavy. Too tired. Too stressed. Too busy. Or too du jour. We tell ourselves that things will change in the future. And when that day arrives, we'll slip off our Oxfords or pumps and lace up our Nikes.

But, unfortunately, that day rarely arrives.

It rarely arrives because "things" in our life rarely change unless we change them. And because the future, by definition, is the offspring of our actions today. To expect a change in the future without instigating that change today is like expecting a flower to blossom from a seed that was never planted. The time to implement change is the present. It's right now.

Too heavy (fat)

You're not alone. Almost 20 percent of runners begin running because they want to lose weight. There's a reason for that: Running, in combination with a smart diet, offers one of the most effective paths for shedding extra pounds. To lose a pound of body weight, you have to burn 3,500 calories more than you eat. While dieting alone can work (fifty million to one hundred million Americans a year give it a try), diets are rarely sustainable (think Christmas, Thanksgiving, birthdays, parties, TV shows, sporting events, late-night snacking, stress snacking, and fast food, not to mention cheese, chips, candy, cookies, cakes, and cream—*and those are just the c's*). That's where running comes in. Running not only burns fat (to the tune of about 75 fat calories per mile), it also helps keep the weight off once you've lost it. That's because running increases the number of calories you can eat each day without putting on weight—both by burning the calories directly and by raising your metabolism for the entire day. And it does this better than other forms of exercise. A 2013 study that followed approximately fifty thousand walkers and runners for six years concluded that running results in 90 percent more weight loss than walking for the same amount of calories burned.

Of course, maybe your concern isn't with losing weight so much as it is with the practicality of running, *period*, at your weight. Maybe you're afraid that you'll ruin your knees (see page 35), or risk a heart attack (see page 38), or damage your body in some other way. You won't. Not if you've gotten your physician's blessing to begin an exercise program and if you follow a smart and sensible training schedule. Or maybe you're worried about being embarrassed, about negative comments people might make or stares you'll get. Again, as we noted in the last chapter, there will *always* be rude and negative people. After I set my first American age-group record, running a 14:45 5K at age forty-five, posters on the running message board letsrun.com variously accused me of being an inattentive parent (since I *obviously* spent too much time training), a performance-enhancing drug user, and probably unemployed—none of which was true. My point is that if people will attack one of the best middle-aged runners in American history, you can expect to hear one or two negative comments no matter *what* you bring to the table. Ignore those comments. Instead, embrace the authentic and heartfelt support you'll receive from family and friends. And, most of all, listen to your inner voice, the one that's reminding you how good it's going to feel to reach your running, fitness, and, yes, weight-loss goals.

Too heavy (large and powerful)

Known as "Clydesdales" in the running world, these runners are taller, wider, more muscular, and bigger-boned (no euphemism) than the stereotypical lean, mean runner-machine. Far from struggling with their greater weight, Clydesdales use their extra muscle to produce more force with each stride. If you're a Clydesdale, you can expect to develop and maintain efficient running form as your fitness improves. And studies show that Clydesdales are no more injury-prone than lighter runners. One accommodation for your weight to consider is buying running shoes with more midsole cushioning. Other than that, happy training!

Too out-of-shape

Really? Isn't this the whole point of starting a running program? Remember that no one starts their program in perfect condition. And no one gets fit in a day. The first day of your program will include only a slight increase in physical activity over the day that preceded it—*and that's it.* You don't even have to run. You can walk. Or do body-weight squats. And then build from there. First, however, you must possess a willingness to try.

Too time-consuming

Yes, it takes time to run. And yes, you're a very busy person. But a running program is time well invested. A 2014 study examining the mortality risks of 55,137 runners and non-runners concluded that running five to ten minutes per day added about three years to runners' lives. So what you give up in time today, you'll get back in spades down the road. And if you increase your running to the twenty to sixty minutes (three to five days per week) recommended by the American College of Sports Medicine, you're still only setting aside the time it takes to watch one TV show, "like" a dozen Facebook posts, or hit the snooze button two or three times in the morning. Assuming thirty minutes of running four times per week, your ability to balance running with the rest of your life amounts to this: balancing the 1 percent of your life you'll spend training with the 99 percent that remains for everything else.

Too tired

Feeling too tired to exercise is quite possibly the *best* reason to start your running program immediately. A 2006 meta-analysis (a review of seventy studies) published in the *Psychological Bulletin* concluded that exercise *increases* feelings of energy and *decreases* feelings of fatigue. And a 2008 study from the University of Georgia estimated that adults who exercise experience a 20 percent increase in energy levels. In addition, a 2006 study, also from the University of Georgia, found that "inactivity is consistently associated with fatigue." In other words, if you're too tired to exercise, it's because you're *not* exercising.

Too stressed

Who isn't? And that's not a good thing. Stress lowers immunity, increases inflammation, slows healing, decreases bone density, decreases muscle mass, increases blood pressure, increases fat, and intensifies blood sugar imbalances. You know what counteracts stress? That's right, running.

Running releases feel-good hormones (the "runner's high"), improves sleep quality, and offers you a daily respite from the pressures of work, family, and other commitments.

Too old

If this is your excuse, you're talking to the wrong person. I've packaged some thoughts on the topic in the sidebar, "Age has nothing to do with it."

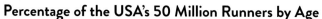

Percentage of the USA's 50 Million Runners by Age

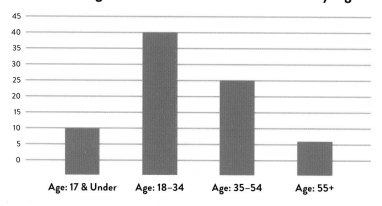

Too hard

As stated previously (and a point to which we'll keep returning), your running program should *never* be too hard. You can only improve incrementally from day to day, so there's never a reason to train harder than necessary to trigger those incremental changes.

Too painful

If by *painful* you mean "fatiguing" or "possibly leading to muscle soreness," see the entry for "Too hard" directly above. If, on the other hand, you're worried about the potential for injuries, such as tendinitis (in its various guises), lower-back stiffness, or muscle strains, read this book's Chapter 12, "Injury Prevention 101," for both a rundown of the different types of injuries and photo instruction for exercises you can do to prevent them.

Too boring

Only if you make it boring. Running is more than the act of putting one foot in front of the other at an accelerated pace. It's the variety of workouts you perform, from runs to resistance training to a ride on an ElliptiGO. It's the places you choose to run, beginning with your neighborhood or local track and then branching out to mountain trails, beach boardwalks, or anywhere your running shoes can carry you. It's the people you run with. The events you enter. And the enjoyment you'll get from achieving your goals. It's the increased energy you'll feel in all your activities. And it's the improved outlook that will follow you throughout the day.

When you postpone a running program because you're *too something*, you miss out on an abundance of *toos* that are intrinsic to the running experience: too healthy, too fit, too happy, too energetic, too confident, and too many new running friends, just to name a few.

EXCUSE CATEGORY TWO: MYTHS

Next up, let's look at a trio of myths that have been used as scarecrows by anti-running alarmists. We've all heard them before, often from a well-meaning family member or friend:

→ "Aren't you worried you're going to ruin your knees?"

→ "Doesn't running damage your heart?"

→ "Don't you worry that you'll get sick running in the rain?"

The answers, in no particular order, are as follows: No, no, and no. For a more comprehensive response, let's tackle these scarecrows one at a time.

Running ruins your knees

No, it doesn't. It does the opposite: It strengthens your knees—*a lot.*

A 2008 Stanford study (referenced in the sidebar, "Age has nothing to do with it") concluded that runners were *seven times* less likely to require knee replacements than non-runners. And a 2013 study on

EXCUSE BUSTER

"Age has nothing to do with it"

So you think you're too old to run?

Just tell that to Stanislaw Kowalski of Poland, who in 2015, at age 105, ran a 100-meter race in 34.50 seconds—into the wind. Or tell it to Hugh Campbell (profiled on page 44), who began running at age eighty-six, then set the American 5K record for ages eighty-five to eighty-nine at 26:33 less than two years later. Or tell Christine Kennedy, who ran a 2:59 marathon at age fifty-nine. Or Ed Whitlock, who recorded a 2:54 marathon at age seventy-three. In fact, the average finisher age in American road races is approximately forty-one years old, leading most road races to include age-group categories, in increments of five to ten years, for runners from their preteens to their eighties.

And not only *can* older potential athletes run, they *should* run.

A 2013 Norwegian study on the health and exercise habits of five thousand people found that your "fitness age" is a better predictor of longevity than your chronological age. Fitness age is based upon a measure of cardiovascular health

osteoarthritis (pain, swelling, and immobility in a joint, especially the knees and hips, caused by loss of cartilage) that followed seventy-five thousand runners and fifteen thousand walkers found that almost twice as many walkers as runners developed the disease—and reported that other non-running exercises provided less protection from osteoarthritis than running, too.

The myth that running hurts your knees springs from the false belief that each foot strike upon the ground must damage bones and cartilage. But it doesn't. In fact, the impact force of each foot strike provides a stimulus that ultimately leads to stronger bones, just as lifting weights leads to stronger muscles. That's why running is better for your knees than walking—because running delivers *more* impact force with each step than walking does.

known as VO2 max. And running is one of the best ways to improve VO2 max. The study concluded that exercise "may significantly improve [muscles, bones,] and overall health, and minimize or delay the effects of aging." It also noted that runners over age fifty typically have a fitness age that is at least twenty years younger than their actual age. To test your own fitness age, use the online calculator at worldfitnesslevel.org/#.

In addition, a 2014 study looked at the impact of running on the heart's left ventricle in more than one hundred people whose average age was seventy. As people age, their left ventricles stiffen, leading to problems ranging from high blood pressure to atrial fibrillation. But the study found that runners who complete four to five workouts per week "throughout adulthood prevent most of these age-related changes." Another 2014 study, conducted by German researchers, concluded that running as we age improves blood flow in our brains, leading to improved memory skills. And a 2008 study from Stanford, which tracked almost one thousand runners and non-runners beginning in 1984, reported that running delays age-related disabilities by almost two decades, reduces the incidence of cancer, reduces the incidence of neurological problems, and reduces health issues related to knees, hips, and the back.

Age isn't a reason not to run; it's one of the best reasons to run that there is.

The bones, ligaments, and tendons that provide your knees' structure are not inorganic matter. Instead, they are living tissue, just like your muscles. When you ignore them, they atrophy—they waste away. When you stimulate them with running, they get stronger.

But what if your knees are already damaged? If you're currently suffering from osteoarthritis, ligament damage, or some other medical condition or injury, you might be justifiably nervous about lacing up your running shoes. For a condition like osteoarthritis, running is actually a part of the treatment (see page 61). For ligament damage and other structural impediments, you'll want to talk to your physician or physical therapist before beginning any fitness routine. But even then, there are loads of exercises—many of which appear in Chapter 12 (see Table 12.1, "Identify Your Running Injury," on page 223)—for overcoming those structural conditions. In any case, the treatment for an already-damaged knee is rarely inactivity; instead, it's therapy, strengthening, and, yes, running.

Bottom line: If you want strong knees, the answer isn't your couch; it's exercise.

Running damages your heart

No, it doesn't. It does the opposite: It strengthens your heart—*a lot*.

I know, I know, you've heard all those stories about marathoners dropping dead mid-race, distance runners developing scar tissue in their hearts, and long-term runners being diagnosed with nasty heart arrhythmias like atrial fibrillation (A-fib). And where there's smoke, there's fire, right?

Wrong.

Here are the facts.

A 2012 study, published in the *New England Journal of Medicine*, tallied the number of heart attacks suffered by 10.9 million competitors in half marathons and marathons between 2000 and 2010. The result was one heart attack for every 184,000 competitors. Fifty-nine total heart attacks, forty-two of them fatal. Put into perspective, that's one fifth of the death rate for triathlons and one sixth that of college athletics.

And a 2013 analysis by the National Runners Health Study, which followed 32,073 runners and 14,734 walkers for six years, found that runners who logged more than twenty-four miles per week had fewer cardiac arrhythmias than those who exercised less (note: We'll specifically address A-fib in "You gotta have heart," page 54).

Runners are 50 percent less likely to experience a serious heart attack than non-runners. That's because running doesn't cause heart attacks. Heart disease causes heart attacks. And what fights heart disease? If you answered, "Running," then congratulations—you've busted this myth.

Running makes you sick

OK, so the answer's not so black-and-white for this one. It's possible for running to lower your resistance to illness, but *only* if you're training at an elite level (i.e., high mileage and high intensity). Otherwise, running improves your resistance to colds and other infections.

Most of us had parents who warned us, at one time or another, that going out in the rain or cold would make us sick. *No, it doesn't.* The viruses and bacteria that cause colds and flu make you sick. And they don't come prepackaged in raindrops and winter breezes. Instead, they congregate on doorknobs, computer keyboards, cell phones, pillowcases, and other surfaces that a sick person has touched. Then you touch those same surfaces, dab your fingers to your mouth, eyes, ears, or nostrils (a UC Berkeley study suggested that we humans touch our faces up to 2,400 times per day), and voilà, you're sick—yet another good reason to wash your hands regularly. It's true that the incidence of colds and flu spikes during fall and winter, but that's not due to weather; instead, it's related to school being in session, people spending more time indoors, lower humidity, and drier mucous membranes in your nose during those months.

What's more, aerobic running *improves* your immune system's ability to fight colds and flu. As Michael Gleeson points out in a 2007 review of research on running and colds, "Regular moderate exercise is associated with a reduced incidence of infection compared with a completely sedentary state." And a 2002 study reported that "risk was reduced by about 20% in men and women [and] was most pronounced in the fall of the year."

So if you're looking for this year's cold and flu season remedy, consider a run.

EXCUSE CATEGORY THREE: ENVIRONMENTAL

When we run out of excuses related to our body and lifestyle, some of us turn to that old standby: the world outside our door. During winter months, we blame the snow, rain, or freezing temperatures. During the summer, we shrink from the heat and humidity. Or maybe it's a precipitous landscape of steep streets and mountain trails that prevents us from heading out the door for a run—or its opposite, pancake-flat roads stretching to the horizon, turning each run into a Sisyphean nightmare during which we seem to get nowhere no matter how long and hard we toil.

But not running because of weather and topography overlooks a fundamental solution available to all runners: When you run, you can create your own environment. By utilizing weather-specific gear (see "Suit Up for Severe Weather," page 73), adjusting the time of day for your workout, and designing exercise sessions with the weather, running route, and your fitness goals in mind, you can create a protective bubble—not unlike an astronaut who dons his or her space suit to walk in outer space.

The heat

Yes, it's tough to run in the heat. But by taking a few precautions, there's no reason you can't join the millions of runners from hot-weather climates who train on a regular basis. Let's start by looking at the two ways your body cools itself when the weather is hot and/or humid: First, if the outside temperature is less than 98.6°F (the average human body temperature), you'll lose heat through *convection* (your blood carries heat to your skin, where it disperses into the air); second, when your sweat evaporates (and it must evaporate for this to work), you lose heat energy. If conditions interrupt either of those mechanisms—if the temperature soars past 98.6°F or the humidity is so high that your sweat doesn't evaporate—you begin to overheat. To combat this, try to run early in the morning or in the evening, when the temperature is cooler and the sun isn't directly overhead. Wear technical fabrics (see Table 5.1), which offer better breathability. Stay hydrated by following the rule: Drink to thirst (drinking too much can lead to other problems). Wear loose outfits, a visor, and sunglasses. Use sunscreen to prevent sunburn. Most important, *slow down*—you'll want to slow your pace ten to fifteen seconds per mile for every 10°F over a perfect (for running) 53°F. If both the temperature and the humidity are high, you won't be able to keep cool. On those days, it's advisable to train indoors (e.g., run on a treadmill in a temperature-controlled room) or take the day off.

The cold, snow, or rain

If cold weather were a legitimate excuse for staying inside, most of the running-gear manufacturers in America would be out of business. With proper cold-weather gear (see Table 5.1), you can run in almost any temperature. In fact, your main challenge will be to avoid *overdressing* for the cold. For rain, there are also good clothing options. With snow, your main obstacle might be terrain—namely, that the terrain is covered by snow. If that's the case, then consider cross training. Both snowshoeing and cross-country skiing are excellent replacement exercises for running.

Hills, hills, and more hills

So we're clear, "hills, hills, and more hills" is actually pretty solid training advice for ambitious runners. But, no, that doesn't mean it's something you want to do every day, especially during the early stages of your running program. Uphill is exhausting. Downhill beats your quadriceps (front thighs) to a pulp. So if you live in a very hilly area, you'll need to drive to an area that's less hilly—a road, trail, or local track—a couple times (or more) per week. Think of it as driving to the gym. On days that you do run hills, don't push the uphills or stride out on the downhills—maintain a consistent effort throughout your run. And by all means, if you have access to a treadmill or elliptical machine, use it once or twice a week.

Flat, flat, and more flat

It's possible to do all your training on flat surfaces. But it isn't optimal. Consider driving to nearby hills once a week. Or if you have a treadmill, set it to an appropriate incline.

Nowhere to run

Runners who live in big cities sometimes face crowded sidewalks, streets that are off-limits, and stoplights every block. Runners in the country might risk their lives on highways with virtually no shoulders. If your area roads aren't conducive to training, you'll have to consider alternatives. Try local high school and college tracks. Or parks. Or off-road trails (hiking paths, fire roads, horse trails, etc.). Or use treadmills or elliptical machines at the gym. If you're simply unsure how or where to plot a course in your area, use MapMyRun (mapmyrun.com) to find a route—there are more than seventy million routes in their database. Or use the USATF database of running routes and tracks (usatf.org/routes).

Or use Google Maps to search for nearby parks and trails. Or just talk to runners; local running stores are a great place to start.

Darkness

Sometimes our schedules force us to run when it's dark. Don't despair. Instead, let there be light. A headlamp (available at most sporting goods stores) will provide illumination—if limited depth perception—for running on roads, sidewalks, or trails with good footing; if you want to improve your depth perception, add a running belt with a built-in light. Many high schools and colleges offer lighted tracks for walkers and joggers in the evening. And most city streets are well lit (residential neighborhoods less so).

Safety

If you're nervous about training in the area where you live, there are a few steps you can take. We'll cover this in far more detail in Chapter 10, but for now:

→ Consider running with a partner.

→ Stick to populated areas.

→ If you're running in the dark, wear bright or reflective clothing, carry a light, and forgo the headphones and music (so you can hear approaching cars and people).

→ Stay aware—stay on the lookout for potholes, head-high branches, cars, strangers, dogs, or any other hazard.

Understanding *everything* about your training environment and preparing appropriately are the keys to making every run a safe, anxiety-free outing.

Right now, as you're reading this line, there are runners everywhere in the USA, and on all four corners of the earth, getting their workouts done. Yes, runners make adjustments for weather, terrain, darkness, and safety. No, one of those adjustments isn't to stop running.

EXCUSE CATEGORY FOUR: THE SIX TO SEVEN INCHES BETWEEN YOUR EARS

All of which leaves us with one last category in this chapter: the stuff that goes on between our ears—specifically, the anti-exercise beliefs that have staked a claim to this six to seven inches and that push the buttons in our personal mission-control center. Of all the excuses documented in this chapter, these are the hardest to overcome. That's because they are often ingrained in the way we think about running. And also because they're the types of excuses that we don't always speak aloud, meaning that they go unexamined in conversation with our family, friends, and acquaintances. So let's try to undo that. Let's discuss aloud what our brains so often attempt to repress.

I hate exercise

Can some of us admit that this is what it comes down to? You hated running that timed mile in eighth grade PE. And nothing you've experienced since has changed your mind. I get it. Not everyone likes to exercise. And if that's all there was to it, if you could spend your life not exercising and remain in recumbent bliss upon the couch, remote control in hand and bowl of Fritos and bottle of beer forever satiating your modest needs, then I'd say go for it. But, unfortunately, that's not the way it works. A sedentary lifestyle is linked to so many serious health problems—including heart disease, cancer, and diabetes—that *Runner's World* dubbed it "the new smoking." And the breakdown in muscle, connective tissue, and nervous system function that accompanies inactivity can eventually make *any* resting position (even sitting) and *any* movement painful. You think exercise hurts? Try knee replacement. Or hip replacement. Or some other disability. Let's step back from the premise of this book for just a moment. Let's forget about getting you into a running program. And let's get real. If you want to remain healthy, active, and independent throughout your life, you'll need to exercise. If you don't like running, then don't. You can walk. Or cycle. Or swim. Or hike, dance, rock climb, ski, golf, kayak, garden, throw a Frisbee, or do anything else that keeps your body rocking. Just. Do. Something.

It takes time away from more important things in life

This excuse isn't about being busy—not really. Everybody is busy. Instead, it comes down to how you view yourself—or, if we're really being honest, how you want other people to view you. It's about the mark you want to leave in the world. It's about keeping your focus on the things that are important in life. If you're like a lot of us, these things include family, work, friends, and community. And maybe a part of you believes

BECOMING A RUNNER: *Hugh Campbell*

Hugh Campbell, age ninety-one, of Glen Mills, Pennsylvania, started running at age eighty-six. By age eighty-eight, he held four American distance-running records (for the eighty-five to eighty-nine age-group). But it wasn't all smooth sailing. "I had problems with my balance when I first started," says Hugh. "I fell a couple times. I fell in one race because I didn't have sense enough to slow down." Hugh also had knee pain. But when his doctor advised him to switch to swimming, Hugh said, "To hell with that." Eventually, the problems got better, and Hugh's running improved. Hugh's decision to become a runner followed twenty-five years during which his only exercise was golf. "I played at least five days a week," he says, "always walking, always carrying my clubs on my back—that's how I kept in shape." During those years, Hugh and his wife, Naomi, lived in a quiet neighborhood in Wilmington, Delaware. "One day, I decided to go for a jog, and then got to where I was jogging pretty good. So I got in the car and measured a three-quarters-of-a-mile loop. I got to the point where I'd do four circuits of that loop. So I decided to run a 5K race." Hugh raced well, and subsequently found himself a targeted recruit for the masters (age forty and over) contingent of his local Pike Creek Valley Running Club. Masters races include an "age-graded" competition, in which each athlete gets a mark based upon the maximum expected performance (which would be "100 percent") for someone his or her age. At age eighty-eight, in Haddonfield, New that it's a little bit selfish to set aside these important things, *for even an hour*, to go running. Again, I get it. But it's an argument with a false premise: that doing one thing (running) negatively affects the others. We all wear many hats in this world. I'm writing this book about running and urging you to become a born again runner like I did, but I'm *not* just a runner. It's not even my most important role. I'm a father. And a writer. And a friend. And a citizen. And a lover of cheeseburgers and candy bars.

Jersey, Hugh ran an American age-group record of 26:33 for 5K, earning a 102.61 percent age grade—the highest 5K mark by a man in American distance-running history. And he did it without any fancy training. "When I joined the club," says Hugh, "they tried to get me to do intervals, but I never had any inclination or patience to do that." A short while after the Haddonfield race, Hugh began to experience pain near the top of his spine. One morning, he couldn't get out of bed. "I had no feeling in my legs," he says. Doctors discovered that a tumor had ruptured and "essentially broken my back." Post-surgery, Hugh had to learn to walk again. Being Hugh, he was soon walking three to four miles at a fifteen-minute-per-mile clip. When his back pain began to return, he capped his outings at a couple of miles with his son—and no faster than twenty minutes per mile. Although his running days have become walking days, Hugh encourages older potential athletes to take up the sport. "Anybody can do it," he says. Asked whether he wishes he'd taken up running earlier in life, Hugh says, "No, I'm delighted. I think my timing was terrific." Anyone looking at his race times would have to agree.

Running doesn't steal from those roles. And it doesn't diminish them. What it does is help me—like it will you—to persevere. Runners take fewer sick days off from work, have more energy, develop fewer psychological disorders (e.g., depression, irritability, and moodiness), suffer less disability (e.g., knee and hip replacements, osteoporosis, and muscular pain), have a reduced incidence of cancer, fewer nervous system disorders, and live an extended life. Yes, there are more important things in life than running. And by running, you'll ensure that you stay healthy enough and live long enough to succeed in all of them.

Fear of failure

We can't leave this chapter without touching on fear of failure. This is a big one. And it's the most basic (and most human) excuse of all. You're afraid to start running because you're afraid you'll fail at running. If you're already struggling with issues like weight, age, or poor self-esteem, the last thing you need is another chance to fail—and to endure the disappointment, anger, sadness, and, most of all, shame that accompanies it. But here's the thing: You won't fail. Not this time. Your body is a physiological machine that is preprogrammed to respond to an exercise stimulus in a very specific and predictable way: It rebuilds itself stronger than before the exercise. The only way you can sabotage that process is by exercising incorrectly. And Part II of this book will make sure that doesn't happen, guiding you through the creation of your own personal action plan.

Excuses aren't a sign of weakness. They're a sign of being human. Letting excuses control your behavior, however, is a different matter. If the obstacles described in this chapter represent the sum total of your resistance to starting a running program, then it's time to lace up the shoes.

On the other hand, there are excuses that go beyond weight, fatigue, pseudoscientific misconceptions, environment, and mere trepidation. These are issues that we can't brush off with a clever paragraph, a personal anecdote, or a few words of encouragement. They are the biomechanical issues that lead to chronic injuries. And medical conditions like heart disease, osteoporosis, and addiction. And they are the subject of the next chapter.

CHAPTER TAKEAWAY

Before many of us can segue from a mental commitment to running to the physical act of stepping out the door, we have to overcome the obstacles that have prevented us from running in the past. When examined closely, most of these obstacles are revealed for what they truly are: excuses. Whether the excuses relate to our physical conditioning (too fat, too tired, too out of shape, etc.), false myths (running ruins your knees), the environment (it's too cold or too hot), or internal roadblocks ("I hate exercise"), most can be easily remedied with accurate information about what a running program entails, the benefits it offers, and the way in which it will fit into your lifestyle. Excuses aren't a reason not to run. Often, they are the *best* reason to run.

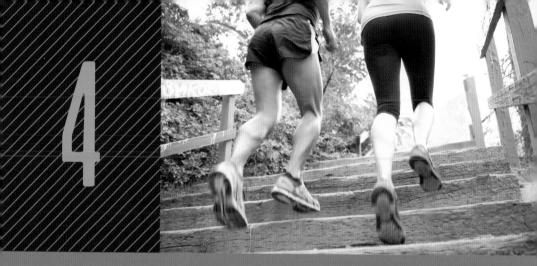

Myth Busting:
The No-Excuse Zone
(Biomechanical and Medical)

"In the depths of winter, I finally learned that within me
there lay an invincible summer."

—ALBERT CAMUS

LAST FOURTH OF JULY, I was at a barbecue, and the topic of running came up. Alex, a young, physically healthy man, shook his head and said, "I don't like running, my body can't handle it." Ashley, his date, an equally young, physically healthy woman, chimed in, "Me, either, it hurts my ovaries." I didn't for a second doubt that Alex and Ashley truly believed what they'd said. They thought running was a bad exercise for their bodies. What I doubted was that they lacked the physical integrity required for running, especially given that they sported the kind of ripped bods that attested to hours in the gym. It was almost certain that Alex and Ashley *could* run. And run very well. It's just that—like Scarecrow, Tin Man, Cowardly Lion, and Dorothy in *The Wizard of Oz*—they had yet to realize that the power to overcome their personal obstacles existed (and had *always* existed) within themselves. They just needed the knowledge and self-confidence to tap into it.

In the last chapter, we tackled excuses of a general nature—the kind that many (maybe most, possibly all) runners peddle at some point. In this chapter, we'll address excuses that relate to specific, tangible concerns you might have for your body or health. We'll start with biomechanical issues, ranging from bad feet to heavy sweating. Then we'll look at medical issues, including heart disease, asthma, and more. Finally, we'll discuss some women's issues, from the above-mentioned "hurts my ovaries" complaint to menstruation and menopause.

It goes without saying that *all runners should consult with their physician before starting a fitness program*—oh, wait, I guess it didn't go without saying. That's because I don't want you to mistake this chapter for a "Get out of seeing your doctor free" card. I want you to overcome the obstacles that have kept you from running, but I also want you to work with your doctor, when applicable, to create a personalized, healthy running program.

EXCUSE CATEGORY FIVE: BIOMECHANICAL

Most "biomechanical" issues are actually this: training mistakes. No one's body is ready to go from zero to 5K (or marathon) training on the first day— or during the first week, or month. That's a recipe for system-wide breakdown, manifested in symptoms such as muscle soreness, shin splints, tendinitis, aching feet, and excessive fatigue.

On the other hand, your body has an amazing capacity for overcoming biomechanical issues. It accomplishes this through *adaptation*, which simply means that your body gets stronger and develops better running efficiency from workout to workout. The caveat is that your body can only accomplish this in incremental bits and pieces. If you're patient, those bits and pieces will begin to add up. And eventually you'll discover that you're sporting a completely *different* body from the one with which you started your program. So before you write off your body as biomechanically deficient, wait until you get a chance to test-drive the new model.

Bad feet

Yes, it's true that flat feet might lead to injury. As might feet with high arches, bumps on the backs of the heels (Haglund's deformity), longer second toes than big toes (Morton's toe), ankle inflexibility, and foot strikes that pronate, supinate, or otherwise deviate from a perfectly prescribed landing. But it's equally true that regularly scheduled resistance training and injury-prevention exercises can mitigate these mechanical challenges (see page 275 to get started); understand, however, that this will require a long-term commitment (think months, not weeks). It's also true that runners with all of these problems are training injury-free right now. That said, if pain and injuries persist, see a podiatrist or sports medicine health professional. They can offer issue-specific counseling and prescribe orthotics (custom-designed shoe inserts) if required. In the meantime, steer clear of generic solutions (e.g., motion-control shoes) that promise results (seldom delivered) for problems (e.g., injuries that result from pronation) that studies can't even prove exist.

Bad form (stride)

The running world suffers from an infestation of form gurus peddling generic form fixes that promise to reduce injuries and improve performance. Some gurus tell you to count strides. Others tell you to let gravity do the work for you. Some warn against using your calves. Or pulling with your hamstrings. Or landing on your heels. Here's my advice: Stop worrying about your form. Large-scale studies consistently find that the most efficient stride is a self-selected stride. A "self-selected stride" is one that develops naturally as the result of long-term participation in a properly constructed running program. In other words, if your form is a problem, it's not because you're biomechanically unfit to run; it's because you're out of shape.

Chronic injury

It's demoralizing. It's depressing. And it's an issue faced by almost all runners who train incorrectly or refuse to include injury-prevention exercises in their schedules. I know. I was one of those runners. And during my four decades of running, I've suffered from Achilles tendinitis, Achilles tendinosis, Achilles bursitis, plantar fasciitis, IT band syndrome, tibial tendinitis, hamstring strains, calf strains, groin strains, sciatica, shin splints, side stitches, back spasms, heat exhaustion, hip pain, knee pain, piriformis syndrome, black toenails, blisters, and five stress fractures in my lower legs. The solution? Simple: a properly designed running program and injury-prevention exercises. Period.

Heavy sweating

Sweating is a good thing. As we mentioned in the last chapter, it's one of two ways in which your body releases heat—when sweat evaporates, you cool down. So the more you sweat, and the more the sweat evaporates, the more you cool your body. Don't fight it. Embrace it.

Lack of flexibility

So you can't touch your toes. So what? Multiple studies show that faster distance runners are *less flexible* than slower runners. A lack of flexibility actually increases your legs' ability to store impact energy with each foot strike (called "elastic energy") and then release it as you push off into the next stride. In layman's terms, you get a free push with each stride! This doesn't mean you should train to be less flexible. You'll want to maintain your natural range of motion for other fitness concerns. But it does mean you shouldn't gripe about not being able to do the splits.

Leg-length discrepancy

I can't tell you the number of runners I've met over the past four decades who've been diagnosed with leg-length discrepancy—a condition in which one leg is shorter than the other. But I can tell you the name of the first person I met who'd been diagnosed with a leg-length discrepancy. Jeff Nelson. He ran for Burbank High School, one of my high school's rivals. In 1979, Jeff ran 8:36 for two miles on the track, a national high school record that would stand for twenty-nine years. So you might say I've been suspicious of leg-length discrepancy as a running obstacle since, well, 1979. It's estimated that between 40 and 90 percent of the population has a leg-length discrepancy. The reason why that estimation covers such a wide range is that the only way to accurately measure leg length is with an X-ray or a CT scan. Getting your bony protrusions felt up in a doctor's office doesn't cut it. Studies have also shown that anything less than a three-quarter-inch (20 mm) difference is inconsequential when it comes to performance or susceptibility to injury, and only one in one thousand people has a discrepancy that large. Even if you do have a significant difference in leg length, the verdict is out on whether heel lifts or raised full-length insoles do you any good. Some people respond well. Some people develop injuries in the foot due to the new biomechanical stresses. So what should you do? Start by recognizing that there's a very good chance your leg-length discrepancy isn't going to be an obstacle. Almost all runners develop strides that compensate for minor discrepancies. Next, include an all-around resistance training program (like the one on page 275) to address muscle imbalances that might be exaggerating the discrepancy (e.g., by causing a lateral pelvic tilt). Finally, if you truly think you have a leg-length discrepancy that's affecting your running, demand that your health care provider accurately measure the discrepancy, account for compensations that occur when you're standing or running, and then, and only then, decide upon a proper course of treatment. In the meantime, heed the findings of a study from way back in 1983: "It is concluded that discrepancies of 5 to 25 mm are not necessarily a functional detriment to marathon runners, and no consistent benefits could be attributed to the use of a lift."

Pelvic tilt

Yes, pelvic tilt—anterior (forward) or lateral (to one side)—can lead to injuries, such as hamstring strains, IT band syndrome, lower back pain, and runner's knee. No, that doesn't mean you can't run. It means you need to strengthen the muscles that control the tilt of your pelvis. For anterior tilt, work your abdominal muscles and incorporate balance exercises. For lateral tilt, strengthen your hip abductors, hip adductors, and hip flexors. Not sure what exercises will help those conditions? No problem. Start with the Beginner's Body Strengthening routine on page 275.

Ran once, now I hurt

If high school running coaches had a dollar for every time a new athlete complained, "I've got shin splints," after the first workout—well, they wouldn't have to work as high school coaches anymore. If you run too hard in your first workout, you *will* hurt. Even if you don't run too hard, you may experience some minor aches and pains. This doesn't mean your body can't run. You're transforming your entire body with your running program. Expect some growing pains.

Biomechanical issues get a lot of attention in the running world. And that attention is usually focused on poor form and bad body parts. There's a reason for that. It's because your stride is something that you can consciously affect—and for which you can implement an immediate change. It's also because physiological conditions like Haglund's deformity and pronation can be seen with the naked eye, and then addressed with tangible fixes—like ice, ACE bandages, and motion-control shoes. In other words, poor form and bad body parts get a lot of attention because snake-oil salesmen can sell you instant, if largely ineffective, "cures." In contrast, you can't see or instantaneously create adaptations to your heart, blood vessels, muscle cells, connective tissue, and nervous system. In a world where we demand and receive instant gratification—from on-demand movies to Amazon's same-day delivery to text messages, online gaming, and even the hookup app Tinder—this inability to see results *now* can seem both antiquated and unacceptable. Yet it is these hidden movers that are ultimately responsible for improved biomechanical function. Biomechanical issues are not excuses to not run. They're your body telling you that you must train smarter.

EXCUSE CATEGORY SIX: MEDICAL

Medical reasons for not running (stop me if you've heard this before— OK, if you've heard it more than a few times before) also tend to be some

EXCUSE BUSTER

"You gotta have heart: Straight talk about running and your heart"

Your heart. It beats one hundred thousand times per day. It pumps your blood through sixty thousand miles of blood vessels. And it delivers oxygen, via twenty to thirty trillion red blood cells, to the one hundred trillion cells in your body. So when something goes wrong with your heart, you're naturally concerned. Correct that. Terrified.

When I was first diagnosed with PVCs (premature ventricular contractions) back in my twenties, I was lucky enough to consult with Dr. Paul Thompson, a cardiologist who practices at Hartford Hospital, about my condition. He explained that in the absence of heart disease or defect, I had nothing to fear. Dr. Thompson has authored more than two hundred articles on the relationship between exercise and the heart, has completed eleven Boston marathons, served as medical commentator for NBC's coverage of the 1988 Olympics, and edited the book *Exercise and Sports Cardiology*. And he agreed to discuss running and the heart for this book.

ARRHYTHMIAS IN RUNNERS

"There are all sorts of arrhythmias," says Dr. Thompson, "and what you should do depends on two things: first, what the arrhythmia is; second, whether you have underlying heart disease—we judge [arrhythmias] based upon the company they keep." If you have an arrhythmia, Dr. Thompson advises talking to a doctor who knows about exercise. If you then get the all-clear (no heart disease, no structural problems), you should be OK to run. Studies back up Dr. Thompson's advice, including a 2015 study published in the *American Heart Journal* that explored whether the stress of a marathon would increase the rate of normally experienced arrhythmias (e.g., nonlethal and isolated incidents of arrhythmia); the study concluded that, for runners who didn't have cardiovascular disease, "the prevalence of arrhythmias during and after a marathon race was decreased." In addition, no malignant arrhythmias (the kind associated with sudden death) occurred.

ATRIAL FIBRILLATION (A-FIB)

Among potential arrhythmias, atrial fibrillation (A-fib), which is an irregular and often rapid heart rate, has drawn attention from runners. Several small studies (not to mention *The Wall Street Journal*) have suggested that long-term running can cause this arrhythmia, which is associated with blood clots and strokes. But Dr. Thompson puts this issue in perspective. "People who exercise the least have the most A-fib," he says. "People who are fit have less of it. And at the highest amounts of exercise, there's a higher rate." But even though elite long-distance runners may experience a higher incidence of A-fib, Dr. Thompson reiterates that lots of people have arrhythmias, and most can run. "If you lie on your left side when you're going to sleep, you'll probably feel a jolt—a skipped beat or a palpitation." That doesn't mean you're dying from an arrhythmia. It just means your heart is normal.

RUNNERS WITH HEART DISEASE

"Most exercise will help people who have prior heart attacks or heart disease," says Dr. Thompson. "You get benefits when you go from being a slug to being a fit person." He points out that this isn't a new idea. In 1768, William Herberden, MD, first identified a new medical condition he called *angina pectoris*. Herberden described angina as a "sense of strangling," accompanied by "anxiety" and pain that sometimes reached the right or left arm. Seeking a potential cure, Herberden described a man who "nearly cured [himself by] sawing wood for half an hour every day." In other words, by exercising. If you do run, Dr. Thompson recommends moderation. "The biggest risk is when people overdo it," he says. "They race too hard or get all crazy with their training. Just have fun running!"

POST-SURGERY RUNNING

For people who have had bypass surgery, received stents, or undergone other surgical procedures for their heart, Dr. Thompson says, "An exercise program will help them. We often have them participate in a cardiac rehabilitation program." Again, he emphasizes, "You don't want to do too much." Still, he's had "lots of patients" who've gone on to finish marathons.

BOTTOM LINE FOR RUNNERS WITH HEART CONCERNS

Dr. Thompson offers these guidelines for runners concerned about a preexisting heart condition:

→ Get a good doctor who is knowledgeable about running and exercise.

→ Diet is very useful, but it doesn't do as much as good medication—so don't fight taking your medications.

→ Don't ignore other risk factors (e.g., high cholesterol, diabetes, blood pressure, etc.).

→ Run for fun, not necessarily to prove anything.

Regarding number four on the list, Dr. Thompson says, "If you're old enough to have heart disease, you're old enough where you don't have to prove anything anymore."

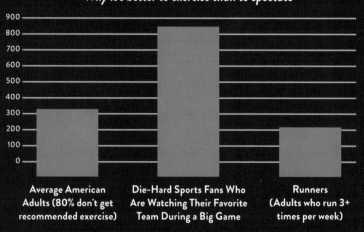

Heart Attacks per Year (per 100,000 Adults)
Why it's better to exercise than to spectate

of the best reasons *for* running. If your body is suffering from the break-down of some tissue or system, strengthening those tissues and systems is usually a good plan. And what's one of the absolute best ways for strengthening those tissues and systems? That's right, running.

Addiction (smoking, drinking, recreational drugs)

I'm listing "addictions" under one heading for two reasons. First, addictions tend to travel in packs. Second, there are so many kinds of addiction—alcohol, street or prescription drugs, tobacco, sex, gambling, food, the Internet, work, etc.—that it'd be impossible to do the topic justice in a running book like this. So instead, we'll start with links to two websites (among many) that offer in-depth information for multiple addictions:

> → **ADDICTIONS AND RECOVERY.ORG:** This website page offers links to recovery groups, self-help forums, treatment locators, government agencies, and other addiction-focused organizations. Visit at: addictionsandrecovery.org/recommended-lists.htm.

> → **HELPGUIDE.ORG:** This site offers information on the signs and symptoms of various addictions, as well as guidance in choosing a recovery program. Visit at: helpguide.org/home-pages/addiction.htm.

Next, you should know that, yes, running *can* play a big role in recovery. Studies have shown that exercise improves recovery from addiction to everything from tobacco to cocaine to morphine. Nora D. Volkow, MD, director of the National Institute on Drug Abuse, has written that exercise "not only boosts energy and keeps weight in check but also helps prevent substance abuse." And an experiment from Simon Fraser University in the 1970s found that rats placed in solitary confinement voluntarily consumed far more "drug solution" than rats allowed to roam "Rat Park," an environment in which the rats could run on wheels, climb, play, and engage in copious amounts of rat hanky-panky. In other words, rats who are allowed to exercise, play, and fool around are less likely to become addicts. While a recovery program is paramount for most addicts, lacing up the Nikes is also a step in the right direction.

Arthritis, fibromyalgia, and lupus

Rheumatoid arthritis (an autoimmune disease causing painful swelling, typically in the small joints of the hands and feet), fibromyalgia (widespread musculoskeletal pain), and lupus (an autoimmune disease that attacks joints, skin, kidneys, blood cells, brain, heart, and lungs) are conditions that might seem to render running off-limits. Not true. According to the Centers for Disease Control: "Scientific studies have shown that participation in moderate-intensity, low-impact physical activity improves pain, function, mood, and quality of life without worsening symptoms or disease severity . . . Both aerobic and muscle-strengthening activities are proven to work well, and both are recommended for people with arthritis." For more information:

→ **Rheumatoid arthritis:** rheumatology.org/Practice/Clinical/Patients/Diseases_And_Conditions/Exercise_and_Arthritis/, and arthritis.org/living-with-arthritis/exercise/how-to

→ **Fibromyalgia:** nchpad.org/160/1203/Fibromyalgia

→ **Lupus:** lupus.org/answers/topic/lupus-and-your-body

Asthma

According to the American Council on Exercise, "The truth is that most asthmatics would likely benefit from some form of regular physical activity." Also, asthmatics who gradually build up their fitness are *less* likely to have attacks during exercise. Like everything in this sport, however, you have to be smart about your approach. Start with these guidelines:

→ Take your time warming up.

→ Keep your running intensity at a moderate level.

→ Take the long view: Slowly improve your fitness over time.

→ Once fit, consider interval training (explained in Chapter 7). The rest periods between repetitions give your lungs time to recover, lessening the chance of serious attacks.

→ Avoid air pollution and cold, dry air.

→ Take your time cooling down.

For more information, visit: acefitness.org/acefit/fitness-fact-article/21/exercise-and-asthma/.

Athletes with disabilities (amputees, spinal cord injuries, cerebral palsy, multiple sclerosis, traumatic brain injury, polio, etc.)

As the aerobic revolution has exploded over the past fifty years, we've come to recognize that *everyone* can benefit from exercise. Athletes with disabilities are no exception. Runners and non-runners alike have become familiar with the sport of wheelchair racing. And South African runner Oscar Pistorius, dubbed the "Blade Runner" by virtue of his two J-shaped carbon fiber prosthetics, made history when he became the first amputee to win a medal (silver) at the world track championships (2011) and to compete in the Olympics (2012). While media coverage of Pistorius's personal life (a murder conviction in 2015) has since eclipsed that of his athletic accomplishments, he helped raise the profile of athletes with disabilities. There are several organizations that offer experienced guidance for athletes with disabilities. Achilles International is a nonprofit organization that provides "a community of support. Able-bodied volunteers and disabled runners come together to train in an environment of support and community. . . . [Runners] gain measurable physical strength and build confidence through their sense of accomplishment." The Wounded Warrior Project offers programs for injured service members. For more information:

→ **Achilles International:** achillesinternational.org

→ **Wounded Warrior Project:** woundedwarriorproject.org/programs/physical-health-wellness.aspx

→ **Amputee:** amputee-coalition.org, amputee-coalition.org/military-instep/introducing-running-lower-limb.html, and completehumanperformance.com/running-amputee

Depression

Here's some good news if you're depressed: Running helps. According to the Mayo Clinic, "Regular exercise probably helps ease depression in a number of ways." Some of these ways include:

→ Running releases "feel-good" brain chemicals that ease depression.

→ It reduces immune system chemicals that intensify depression.

→ It increases body temperature, which can have a calming effect.

→ It takes your mind off negative thoughts.

→ It creates the opportunity for social interaction.

→ You practice a healthy coping strategy.

→ Achieving running goals helps you gain confidence.

Diabetes

Whether you have type 1 diabetes or type 2 diabetes, the American Diabetes Association (ADA) states that "regular physical activity is important for your overall health and fitness." The ADA recommends aerobic exercise (e.g., walking and running), strength training, flexibility exercises, and balance exercises. Lucky for you, all four of those recommendations are part of the training outlined in Part II of this book. The Centers for Disease Control echo the ADA, suggesting a regimen of "moderate-intensity physical activity for at least 30 minutes on 5 or more days of the week." And the American Council on Exercise lists the following advice for runners with type 2 diabetes (90 to 95 percent of all diabetic cases):

→ Consult your physician before starting your running program.

→ Try to burn a minimum of 1,000 calories per week. Increase this to 2,000 calories for weight loss.

→ Do resistance training at least twice per week.

→ Perform stretching exercises 2–3 times per week.

For more information, try the following links:

→ **Publication:** "What I Need to Know About Physical Activity and Diabetes": niddk.nih.gov/health-information/health-topics/Diabetes/physical-activity-diabetes/Pages/physical-activity-diabetes.aspx

→ **American Diabetes Association:** diabetes.org

→ **CDC on Diet**: cdc.gov/diabetes/living/eatright.html

→ **Tips from the Mayo Clinic:** mayoclinic.org/diseases-conditions/diabetes/expert-blog/insulin-and-exercise/bgp-20056553

Heart Disease

Heart disease is covered in "You gotta have heart: Straight talk about running and your heart" (page 54).

Osteoarthritis

More than twenty-seven million Americans suffer from osteoarthritis—the most common form of arthritis, causing pain, swelling, and reduced motion in the joints, including the knees, hips, hands, and spine. According to the National Institutes of Health (NIH), "exercise is one of the best treatments for osteoarthritis. . . . [And exercise], if done correctly, has few negative side effects." As a personal aside, one of my clubmates, Ken Ernst, was diagnosed with osteoarthritis of the knee at age forty-nine. He was advised to quit running. One year later, at age fifty, Ken set the American record for 5000 meters (5K on a track) for ages fifty to fifty-four with a 15:34 performance. Four years later, he's still running strong. For more information, visit: niams.nih.gov/Health_Info/Osteoarthritis/default.asp#7.

Osteoporosis

Osteoporosis is covered in "The bare bones: Straight talk about running and osteoporosis" (page 64).

Visual impairment

Not only is it possible to run, train, and compete with visual impairment, but Marla Runyan, a distance runner who is legally blind, won three USA national championships at 5000 meters, won national road race championships at 5K and 10K, competed in two Olympics (2000 and 2004), and was the top American woman at the 2002 New York City Marathon, running 2:27:10. Marla's advice for runners with visual impairment, as conveyed in an interview with *Vision Loss Resources*, is to find someone who can show—not *tell*—you how to perform. "You need to meet with the [person with visual impairment] and say, look, you can do this, I am going to show you how." Many runners with visual impairment choose to run with a guide. Guides can offer verbal direction or can assist through the use of a tether (a short length of rope or towel held by both guide and runner). For more information on guides or on organizations that provide assistance to runners with disabilities, visit:

→ **American Foundation for the Blind:** afb.org/info/living-with-vision-loss/recreation/running-2805/235

→ **Achilles International:** achillesinternational.org

Wears glasses

So do millions of active runners. Many wear their normal glasses while running, but most opt for contact lenses. Some runners train in their glasses and then race in contact lenses. Still others run "blind," leaving the glasses at home. A few other tips include:

→ Because brightness can be amplified by glasses, some runners choose prescription sunglasses.

→ A more common choice to combat brightness is to pair contact lenses with running sunglasses (e.g., Oakleys).

→ When it rains, a hat or visor can help keep raindrops off your lenses.

→ Use your shirt to clear away condensation on cold or muggy days.

When I asked glasses-wearing Peter Gambaccini, an online journalist for *Runner's World*, for his take on the subject, he reflected that "glasses protect me from unexpected attacks by flying creatures and objects." He added that he once beat "a very revered runner in a track race. His friend, within earshot of me, asked him, 'How could you let that Clark Kent dude beat you?' That was a career highlight, not so much as a runner but as a Clark Kent dude."

EXCUSE CATEGORY SEVEN: JUST FOR WOMEN

For our final excuse category, let's turn to a few of the remaining challenges that women face. Of course, most of these aren't excuses. They're biological realities that must be addressed. The good news is that approximately twenty-five million women are already jogging and running, so the chance that any of these issues will hold you back is virtually nonexistent.

Breasts

Yes, you have them. So, yes, you'll need a sports bra. There are sports bras for every shape and size. There are compression bras, which use a solid band of tight, stretchy fabric to hold breasts in place. And there are encapsulation bras, which provide a separate cup for each breast. For more information on picking the right sports bra for you, visit:

→ **"Sports Bras: How to Choose":** rei.com/learn/expert-advice/sports-bras.html

→ **"Your Sports Bra Fitting Guide":** fitnessmagazine.com/workout/gear/sports-bras/how-to-choose-a-sports-bra

Menopause

Millions of female runners are either dealing with menopause or will have to confront it in the future. Its challenges include hot flashes, sleep problems, mood changes, weight gain, and slowed metabolism, among others. The good news is that running can improve both your mental and physical outlook during menopause. A 2014 Finnish study found that physically active women undergoing menopause "showed higher quality of life" than inactive women. And a 2012 study concluded that "well-being is not associated with menopausal status per se but is associated with current health status." The study suggested that "menopause may be a window of opportunity, since it may induce lifestyle modification." And while issues such as cardiovascular disease, osteoporosis, and urinary incontinence affect post-menopausal women, top age-group sprinter Liz Palmer, now

EXCUSE BUSTER

"The bare bones: Straight talk about running and osteoporosis"

More than fifty-three million Americans age fifty and older suffer from osteoporosis or osteopenia. That number is expected to rise to sixty-four million by 2020 and seventy-one million by 2030. Osteoporosis occurs when old bone is broken down by your body (a natural process) faster than it is replaced with new bone. This leads to low bone density and an increased chance of fractures—bending over or coughing can lead to a break. Osteopenia occurs when bone density is below normal, but not low enough to be diagnosed as osteoporosis. Osteoporosis causes 1.5 million fractures in the United States every year. While osteoporosis strikes both genders, it's especially prevalent among postmenopausal women, with some studies estimating up to a 10 percent loss of bone mass in women during the first five years after menopause.

Running and resistance training have both proven effective for maintaining bone density. But runners already diagnosed with osteoporosis and osteopenia have a legitimate concern about potential fractures. Dr. Aurelia Nattiv, director of the UCLA Osteoporosis Center and the team physician for the UCLA Department of Intercollegiate Athletics, answered a few questions about running with low bone density.

Is it safe to run with osteopenia or osteoporosis?
"For those with osteopenia, running can be good for their bones, as long as it's not in excess—to the point that the person is in a chronic energy deficit," says Dr. Nattiv. "For those with osteoporosis, it's a good idea to check with your physician to make sure the types of exercise you are doing are bone beneficial."

What factors should be considered when determining whether it's safe to run?
"Risk factors such as age, overall health, prior fractures, bone density, menstrual periods, family history of osteoporosis, BMI, medications, and other health conditions should be assessed prior to determining if running is safe. . . .

Also, some individuals may be able to run short distances, but not long distances or excessive mileage, depending on their bone density and risk factors."

Is running a treatment for the disease?

"For low bone mass, some running or a walk/jog can certainly be bone beneficial. However, high-intensity running for long distances can be harmful in some individuals with osteoporosis, especially if untreated. Running itself in a postmenopausal female with osteoporosis will usually not be enough to improve bone density, but it can help in conjunction with vitamin D, calcium, and osteoporosis medications if needed."

If running isn't safe, what exercise is recommended?

"Walking is OK for most people, unless they have pain with this mode of exercise. Jogging may be too strenuous for some. In addition, strengthening exercises are bone beneficial—such as Pilates, yoga, or weight lifting with light weights. The strengthening can help balance, which is important for fall prevention."

Are there medications to strengthen bones for running?

"It's a combination of exercise, bone-building nutrients—vitamin D, calcium, and others—and medications in those with osteoporosis that can help strengthen bone. In some with osteoporosis, it is feasible to jog, but it's usually not the medicine alone that will determine this."

What's the danger for runners with osteoporosis?

"The dangers are running excessively beyond what their physician recommended, not replenishing their energy [calories] to meet the demands of their exercise, and running too strenuously to the point of bone fatigue and possible fracture."

The World Health Organization has created an online tool for predicting your personal ten-year risk of suffering a fracture related to osteoporosis. To use it, go to: shef.ac.uk/FRAX.

Gideon Connelly, age twenty-five, of Tampa, Florida, was twenty-one years old when he lost control of his 2003 Yamaha R1 motorcycle. "I had a funny feeling that day," says Gideon. "I thought I shouldn't get on the bike. But I did it, anyway." When the Yamaha's throttle stuck, Gideon tried to pop the clutch, to get the bike out of gear. "As I did, the bike slid out on its rear wheel." The bike flipped, throwing Gideon onto a curb. A fraction of a second later, the bike came down on Gideon's leg. "I tried to stand up," says Gideon, "and I realized my foot was missing, my right knee was snapped in half, and my arm was bent backwards the opposite way." Gideon was a crew chief for the A-10 in the Air National Guard, so he was eventually transferred to Walter Reed National Military Medical Center. "The doctors were trying to save my leg," he says, "to regrow the bone and fuse my foot to my tibia." When that didn't work, Gideon made the decision to amputate the leg. "It hit me hard," he says. "I'd been into bodybuilding and looking my best all the time. I was vain." But as Gideon observed other service members arrive at Walter Reed, many far worse off than he, his mind-set changed. "I made the choice that I wasn't going to give up, and I was going to pursue my life without my leg." Gideon hadn't run since his freshman year of high school, but he decided to try again. He found a running prosthetic, engaged a coach, and began training. Not that there weren't a few bumps in the road. "I got my first prosthetic the day before Thanksgiving," says Gideon, "and then walked around the whole next day. I bruised my leg to the point where I couldn't put my prosthetic back on." Once healed, Gideon brought

fifty-four, offers this motivational observation: "Once you're on the other side, you no longer have to deal with the regular hormonal fluctuations that you had before menopause—everything has stabilized!"

Menstrual cycle

First, the challenging news. During your menstrual cycle, you'll experience large fluctuations in hormones, changes in energy usage (burning fat and sparing carbs), bloating, the potential for athletic anemia, increase in body temperature, cramping, and other issues. The good that same determination to his workouts. He learned to sync the "return" he got from his prosthetic and good leg. Practiced driving his knee to his chest, rather than whipping his prosthetic to the side. And, finally, he raced. First, at the Texas Regional Games. Then at the Endeavor Games. He increased his training to four times per week and started running faster. He eventually participated in the Wounded Warrior Games (woundedwarriorproject.org), where he ran alongside fellow service members with disabilities, making five "really good friends," all of whom now sport matching tattoos. Connelly trains hard to inspire other runners with disabilities. "Once people see that they can do something," he says, "then they can go for it." He steers potential athletes to YouTube. "There are a million people with disabilities [on YouTube] who are out there inspiring people. Find one, look them up on Facebook or wherever, and that will link you to other people. There's so much potential for what you want to attain."

news is that millions of women have already shown that you can run anyway. As Tania Fischer, coach of the two-time women's national cross country champion team the Janes recently told me, "You can run on your period—it isn't going to make it worse, and, in fact, you feel better most of the time since you're getting fresh air and moving your body." For two good articles on the topic, visit:

→ **"Running Around the Menstrual Cycle":** running.competitor. com/2014/03/training/running-around-the-menstrual-cycle_67117

→ **"How Menstruation Affects Your Running":** runnersworld.
com/rt-web-exclusive/how-menstruation-affects-your-running

Pelvic Pain (females)

Yes, as noted in this chapter's opening paragraph, pelvic pain can be caused by a problem with the ovaries. Many women have ovarian cysts without knowing it, and this can cause pain during exercise. Also, ovaries (like testicles in men) are subject to bouncing during runs, which can lead to pain and require some type of support. Pain can also be "referred" from a nearby organ, muscle, or ligament, in which case the prescription is core training, rest, or (again) abdominal support. Another trigger for pelvic pain is dehydration, which leads to cramping. If you're experiencing pelvic pain, you'll want to check with your doctor. But chances are you've got a condition that can be treated, and you'll be back on the roads in no time.

No experienced running coach would suggest that biomechanical and medical issues shouldn't be treated seriously. They should. It's just that "treated" is the operative word. The miracle of running is that it can improve both biomechanical and medical issues that, left to themselves, would remain as they are or get worse. If you respect your body, you'll do what it takes to improve your body. But the key word, as it has been and will remain throughout this book, is *patience*. It will take time. And it will take self-confidence. And, most of all, it will take that first step out the door—which begins with the very next chapter.

CHAPTER TAKEAWAY

Biomechanical and medical issues create real obstacles for many runners. That's the bad news. The good news is that most biomechanical issues stem from training mistakes—or, at least, from the absence of a smart full-body running program. And most medical issues can actually be improved with running; if they can't, there are usually program modifications that can make running possible. The bottom line is that, for every biomechanical or medical issue, running isn't a problem; it's part of the solution.

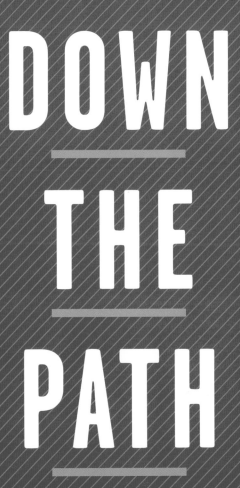

PART TWO

DOWN THE PATH

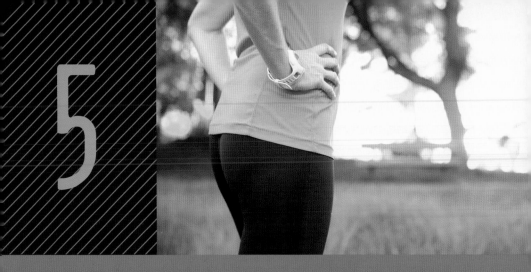

Run First, Train Later

"The river swells with the contribution
of the small streams."
—BATEKE PROVERB

OK, SO YOU'RE READY TO RUN—or to walk, lift weights, or perhaps get your program rolling with a little cross training. You're poised at the threshold. You just need some advice on what, exactly, to do once you step out the door.

And here it is: Run first, train later.

Anyone who's watched a toddler learn to walk understands that control of leg movement and balance is not instinctive. It's a learned skill. Hundreds of bumps and boo-boos by the time each of us reached age two attest to as much.

It's the same with running. Your muscles and bones and tendons aren't ready to run. Your nervous system isn't wired to produce an efficient stride. Your fuel supplies are low. Your balance is underdeveloped. And your brain's ability to gauge effort and fatigue is raw.

Trying to train at this point—to string together challenging work-outs with the objective of transforming your body to meet a specific, predetermined goal—is just silly. You have no idea what your body is capable of doing. No idea whether you can sustain a run. Or walk for more than a few minutes without collapsing into a mound of quivering Jell-O. In fact, the only thing you absolutely *do* know right now is that you haven't been running, which, in the world of reality-based fitness planning, means *you're not ready to train.* Training now would be like setting sail in a boat with a sputtering bilge pump, leaky hatch, cracked hoses, and improper wiring—yeah, you'd probably clear the harbor, but, yeah again, it wouldn't be long before you sank.

What you *are* ready to do is to fortify your running body. And, if all goes well, to do a little bit of actual running. So that's where you'll begin. You'll strengthen your muscles, bones, and tendons. Rewire your nervous system for better control of your stride. Expand the fuel capacity of your muscle cells. And become familiar with your body's feedback while exercising. If all of that sounds intimidating, I can promise you that, in practice, it won't be. No one's asking you to consciously address each of the above objectives—to delve into the intricacies of anatomy, physiology, and exercise science. Instead, you'll use a combination of simple exercises and equally simple exercise strategies to awaken your body, stimulate the desired improvements, and become familiar with the sensations accompanying increased physical activity, the physical demands of exercise (e.g., movement and balance), and the first inkling of fatigue.

In doing so, you'll avoid the first (and biggest) mistake that runners make, the one that dooms up to 80 percent of new running programs: You try to train hard from day one with a body that's not even ready to run.

This chapter will guide you through your very first workout. And then your first few weeks. Along the way, you'll learn some basic running terms, but nothing that will make your head spin, I promise. Learning basic terminology isn't about becoming a running expert. It's about understanding concepts that will help you make informed workout decisions.

Our goal during these initial weeks is to arm you with a stronger, more efficient, and more energetic runner's body. Once that's accomplished, you'll be ready to train.

SUIT UP!

First things first. You'll need to get dressed.

In Chapter 2, we introduced a guiding principle, "Shirts, shorts, shoes," that advised against over-shopping for your initial running gear. That advice still stands, with one big exception: If you live in an area subject to severe weather, you'll need to add a few items to your list. Yes, I know, some of you are tough and can handle anything Mother Nature throws your way. But, in running, toughness isn't about individual acts of stoicism (e.g., an all-out effort in subzero temperatures wearing nothing but skivvies that lands you on the couch—or in the hospital—the next day). In running, toughness is defined by long-term perseverance, by notching workout after workout, week after week, month after month.

And one way to ensure that perseverance is to control your current workout environment. Running when you're too cold, too hot, or too wet may seem like a doable challenge for a day or two, but after a week—or a month—it can become a program killer. With that in mind, visit Table 5.1 for some practical advice on accessorizing for weather.

> **LEARNING TO LAUGH AT OURSELVES**
>
> "First clue you're not getting enough exercise: Your dog is fat." —Unknown

IT FEELS LIKE THE FIRST TIME

Everyone gets excited for their first run. Doesn't matter whether it's your *first* first run or just your first run back after a break. It's a new beginning. A time for optimism. A physical manifestation of "looking forward" rather than remaining mired in the past.

But it's also this: the workout that sabotages more running programs than any other.

Your first workout isn't the time to test out your body's current fitness level. We already know what that level is. You're *out of shape*. Run

Suit Up for Severe Weather

Technical Fabrics—Wick away excess moisture while still allowing sweat on skin to evaporate (essential to cooling) • Provide good breathability

Loose Shorts—Allow better breathability • Longer shorts provide better sun protection

Hat with a Brim or Visor—Protects your face from the sun • Cotton caps (e.g., baseball caps) can trap heat; look for technical fabrics

Sunglasses—Protect your eyes • Reduce stress

Sunscreen— Protects your skin from the sun

Handheld Water Bottle—Hydrates

RAIN

Zippered Jacket or Vest—Can be adjusted when the rain starts or stops • The zipper can be used as a thermostat

Tights or Pants—Those with a waterproof panel in front will shield you from the rain

Technical Running Socks—Are good for any run, but especially in the rain (you'll have drier feet, and your socks won't shift inside your shoes) • Cotton socks are a recipe for blisters • Merino wool keeps your feet warmer and resists odor

Hat with a Brim—Keeps the rain off your face

SNOW & EXTREME COLD

First Layer—A synthetic layer (technical fabric) next to the skin, to wick away moisture

Second Layer—An insulation layer; a half-zip design, buoyed by some spandex, works great

Third Layer—A windproof jacket (a shell to cover your other layers); should have zippers under the arms or full-length to serve as your thermostat

Underwear—Non-cotton; men should look for underwear with a windproof panel (trust me!)

Tights—Classic tights, with a polyester-and-spandex blend

Running Pants—Less clingy than tights; can be used as second layer or as third layer (over tights) when it's freezing

Hat—Merino wool

Gloves or Mittens—Built-in, fold-over mittens

Shoes—A hybrid trail shoe with a Gore-Tex-type upper, to keep your feet warm and dry

ALTITUDE

Hydration Belt or Water Bottle—You'll get dehydrated at altitude faster than at lower elevations Pick a hydration belt that sits low on your hips and doesn't bounce around (belts that ride up can put pressure on your belly and leave you nauseated)

Sunscreen—You get an 8-10% increase in sun intensity for every 1,000 feet in gained elevation too hard, even for a single workout, and your body will break. You'll end up incapacitated by DOMS or a more serious issue.

Instead, you should rein in your excitement and treat this first workout like a multivitamin. You don't try to swallow a vitamin pill better and faster than anyone has ever swallowed a pill before. Same goes for your first workout. This isn't the time for performing an exercise routine that could be seamlessly edited into the original *Rocky* film (somewhere between drinking raw eggs for breakfast and ascending the steps of the Philadelphia Museum of Art, hands held high in triumph). It's the time to do the workout. Period.

If you want to celebrate afterward, go for it. Enter your workout into a training log. Down a recovery drink. Play inspirational music. High-five family members and friends (or, better yet, a training partner). Your mind will be on fire with the significance of this huge step forward in your life. Just make sure your legs aren't on fire, too.

Step one: Make the time

You'll need to set aside thirty to sixty minutes for your first workout. Even if you're only going to be exercising for a few minutes (e.g., a five-minute walk), you'll need time to get dressed, do the workout, perform some post-workout exercises, and then shower.

While you're at it, pick at least three times a week when you can do the same, and make sure to schedule at least one recovery day between workout days. If you're planning on four or more workouts per week, some workouts will have to occur on back-to-back days. If that's the case, try to spread both workouts and recovery days evenly throughout the week.

Do *not* just play it by ear when it comes to setting aside time for workouts. You had a busy schedule already. Don't expect hour-long free periods to magically materialize now that you're running.

Step two: Choose your first workout

Which brings us to the question: *What, exactly, should you do for a first workout?*

You got a book about running. So you probably opened this book with the expectation that you'd be running from day one. By now, however, I'm guessing you've figured out that a running program is about a lot more than "running." So while your goal is absolutely to become a practicing runner, the quickest route between here and there might not begin with a run. It might begin with an easy walk. Or some walking with jogging surges. Or, if you're pretty fit (from previous non-running exercise), some walking with longer jogging surges.

There are a few things to take into consideration:

1 **CURRENT FITNESS:** You'll need to honestly appraise your current fitness. If you've already been active (e.g., going on walks, playing pickup basketball, etc.), then you'll be ready for a little more work on day one. If you've been completely inactive, you'll have to start less ambitiously.

2 **HEALTH ISSUES:** If you have any of the health issues discussed in the previous two chapters—from weight issues to asthma to heart disease—then you'll want to be extra cautious with your initial outings.

3 **WEATHER:** You don't want to perform your first workout in a blizzard. Or in a virtual sauna. If severe weather conditions are present, you'll want to take your workout indoors, where you can begin with resistance training or, if the equipment is available, aerobic cross training. (When you've improved your fitness to the point where you're confident that you can perform the scheduled exercise, that's the time to suit up and face the extra challenge of severe weather.)

Once you've assessed the above criteria, it's time to get specific. Table 5.2 offers some examples of first workouts. Some of you will want to do more than the suggested exercise. In response, I'd ask, *Why?* Your goal is to be running a few months down the line. A bigger first workout won't get you there faster. It will only increase your chance of injury. Your primary objective right now is to build a body that *can* run. Remember, training comes later.

First Workout*

Definition: You don't have an exercise base. You spend most of the day seated, and the walking you do is limited to small excursions around the house or to and from your car.

Good Weather: 10–15 minutes of easy walking

Good Weather (health issues): 5–10 minutes of easy walking

Bad Weather: One set of each exercise from the Beginner's Body Strengthening routine (page 275)

Bad Weather (access to treadmill, elliptical trainer, or other): Same volume (time) and intensity as good weather

ACTIVE (WITH NO TRAINING BASE)

Definition: You don't participate in a fitness program, but you still use your legs to get around (e.g., you walk or bicycle at least part of the way to work, you play golf, etc.) and/or are active at your job or around the house (e.g., gardening, construction projects, etc.)

Good Weather: 10–20 minutes alternating easy walking with 10- to 15-second surges of jogging

Good Weather (health issues): 10–15 minutes of easy walking

Bad Weather: One set of each exercise from the Beginner's Body Strengthening routine (page 275)

Bad Weather (access to treadmill, elliptical trainer, or other): Same volume (time) and intensity as good weather

ACTIVE (WITH TRAINING BASE)

Definition: You've been participating in some type of fitness routine—walking, cycling, weight lifting, pickup basketball, etc.—and feel that just walking would be a step backward in your fitness program.

PLANNING WEEKS 1 THROUGH 3 (OR MORE)

With the first workout under your belt, it's time to look ahead to the next few weeks. Just as you chose a day one workout that matched your fitness, health, and environment, you'll want to schedule a manageable

Good Weather: 10–20 minutes alternating easy walking with 1- to 3-minute surges of jogging

Good Weather (health issues): 10–20 minutes alternating easy walking with 10- to 15-second surges of jogging

Bad Weather: One set of each exercise from the Beginner's Body Strengthening routine (page 275)

Bad Weather (access to treadmill, elliptical trainer, or other): Same volume (time) and intensity as good weather

RETURNING RUNNER (INJURED)

Definition: You ran in the past for an extended period of time, achieving a level of fitness that you'd either like to recapture or surpass.

Recommendation: See all above categories, then start with the one that matches your current activity level. While you can expect to progress more quickly than a newbie to the sport, that progression will show up in the weeks to come—not on day one.

RETURNING RUNNER (CHRONIC INJURIES)

Definition: You ran in the past for an extended period of time, achieving a level of fitness that you'd either like to recapture or surpass. But you've been dogged by chronic injuries (likely developed while running in the past) and don't want to begin a new program that will be hobbled by the same physical setbacks.

Recommendation 1: See all above categories, then start with the one that matches your current activity level. While you can expect to progress more quickly than a newbie to the sport, that progression will show up in the weeks to come—not on day one.

Recommendation 2: Incorporate—from day one—both the Beginner's Body Strengthening routine (page 275) and any injury-specific exercises from the Injury-Prevention Exercises (page 224) that relate to your chronic condition.

* Always consult with a physician, dietitian, or other health care professional before beginning or making any changes to an exercise program or diet.

workload for this crucial period. After Chapter 6 (look for the blue-colored band in the middle of this book), you'll find this book's "Training Schedules," which offer sample schedules that cover both the first few weeks of your program and the weeks that follow. You can implement one of these schedules as written, or you can alter it to fit your specific goals and preferences. Regardless of which option you choose, you'll want to understand a few key concepts that guide the creation of a practical and effective schedule—concepts like mileage, minutes, intensity, and listening skills. In plotting out an incremental progression in your schedule (a process that begins on day one), it's important to understand how to measure your exercise volume, as well as how to recognize when it's time to alter that volume. These aren't the kinds of science-y concepts that only exercise scientists and elite coaches are required to master. Instead, they're everyday topics that runners routinely discuss. Understanding them will help you to make smart workout decisions.

Mileage

Mileage is both a popular and a simple way for runners to keep track of their running volume. Your mileage is the total number of miles you accumulate during a week's worth of workouts. If you walk or run one mile, three times per week, your mileage is three miles (1 x 3 = 3). If you walk or run three miles, five times per week, your mileage is fifteen miles (3 x 5 = 15). Mileage includes the total distance you walk, run, and race during a week (including all distance covered during warm-ups and cool-downs—also called warm-downs).

Most runners focus on "mileage" when creating a running program. At group workouts and races, you'll often hear runners comparing their mileage with one another. In fact, "What's your mileage?" pretty much serves as the running world's communal greeting.

Runners who use mileage as the basis for their running programs believe that physiological benefits accrue with increased mileage. In other words, they believe that running thirty miles per week will make them fitter than running fifteen miles per week. And that sixty miles per week is better than thirty.

There's only one problem with relying solely upon "mileage" when creating a running program: Mileage is an extraordinarily inaccurate way to measure the actual workload of your program, as you'll see next.

Minutes

Another way to calculate your workload is to measure your exercise volume by minutes. With this method, you don't count the miles you cover during walks and runs. Instead, you count the total minutes you spend exercising.

If you think about it, it's pretty obvious why minutes are better than miles when outlining your workout schedule. Let's say you have two runners, Runner A and Runner B. And let's say that Runner A trains at six minutes per mile on distance runs, and the less-fit Runner B trains at twelve minutes per mile. At those paces, it will take Runner B twice as long as Runner A to run one mile. That means that if both runners try to log the same mileage, Runner B will have to run twice as many minutes as Runner A! Do we really think that a less-fit runner should be running twice as long as a fit runner?

The answer is "No." Slower runners shouldn't be training longer than faster runners. What's more, to achieve the same fitness stimulus relative to their ability, they don't have to. In running, you improve based upon the amount of time you spend exercising at specific effort levels. If a fast runner logs thirty minutes, he or she gets thirty minutes' worth of training stimulus. If a slow runner logs thirty minutes, he or she *also* gets thirty minutes' worth of training stimulus. Doesn't matter if the fast runner covers five miles (six-minutes-per-mile pace) and the slow runner covers two-and-a-half miles (twelve-minutes-per-mile pace). As far as their bodies are concerned, it's the same workout.

In this book, we'll use "minutes" when discussing the length of walks and runs.

Intensity

Intensity refers to how hard you exercise during a workout. Walking and jogging are low-intensity workouts. An all-out run is a very high-intensity workout. Workouts such as distance runs, repetitions, hill running, and plyometrics occupy intermediate rungs on the intensity ladder—don't worry if you aren't familiar with all those types of training, as they'll be explained in Chapter 7. When you increase the intensity of a workout, you create a harder workout, and you also create the need for more recovery time afterward.

And therein lies another problem with basing your running program on mileage.

Mileage doesn't take intensity into account. If you design a program based on mileage, then a mile of walking is equivalent to a mile of uphill sprints. Only it's not. The walking is a low-intensity workout that will require very little recovery time (maybe a day, at most). The sprinting is an extremely high-intensity workout that both damages muscle cells and exhausts your nervous system—it will be days before you're ready to challenge your body again.

It's especially important to take intensity into consideration when planning your first workouts. That's because *every* workout at the beginning of a running program is "intense" as far as your body is concerned. Until you've done some basic strengthening, you won't want to risk any type of higher-intensity training. For instance, fifteen minutes of continuous walking is manageable for most people at the start of their running programs, but fifteen minutes of continuous running is not.

Determining correct exercise volume and intensity

So how much should you exercise during your first few weeks? And how hard?

The answers, respectively, are: Not much, and not very.

For your first few weeks, excessive fatigue is not on the menu. You'll want to schedule incremental increases in exercise volume and intensity (we'll discuss how to determine these increases in a minute), but you'll *never* want to reach a point where you "feel the burn." *Feeling the burn* makes for good fitness product advertisements, but in the real world it also makes for injured, burned-out, and sidelined runners.

Pain and fatigue are your body's way of telling you that you're overloading your systems. *Listen to your body.* Pay attention to its feedback. Your body won't lie to you. If your body says, "Hey, this is too hard for me," believe it.

There will be a time for pushing through fatigue in your running program.

Now is not that time.

Developing listening skills

Instead, now is the perfect time to develop improved communication between your mind and body—the art of "listening to your body" (referenced above). As you begin to incorporate the elements of an all-around running program, your mind will learn to process the signals being sent by your body during exercise. You will learn to recognize and respond to:

→ Physiological changes in your body as you warm up

→ Insufficient energy levels (due to inadequate diet, poor sleep, or high stress)

→ Problems with your stride

→ Increasing or decreasing rate of breathing, and its relationship to effort level

→ Twinges in joints that are forerunners to more serious injuries

→ Heaviness in your arms and shoulders as an indication of impending fatigue

→ Muscle discomfort when your pace exceeds your target effort level

→ Anxiety or lethargy as a sign of overtraining

→ . . . and much more

Of course, you'll be a long way from mastering that level of body awareness on your first day. On that day, you might very well believe that your body is speaking a foreign language—and that your legs are having an equally hard time processing the instructions you're sending from your brain. Don't worry. This is normal. It takes time to develop an efficient mind-body connection. But by honing your listening skills now—by sharpening your ability to process all the sensations that occur during exercise—you will soon become fluent in your body's language. When you progress to harder training in the months to come, this skill will be invaluable. You'll detect the first inkling of injuries long before they occur. Will learn to anticipate dehydration and energy bonks. And will recognize in advance when it's necessary to ease off your running to avoid overtraining—a mistake (see Chapter 8, page 152) that can set your program back months.

Increasing exercise volume and intensity

During these first few weeks, you won't schedule major increases in either volume or intensity. That's because exercising at all is a *huge* increase over your previous state of not exercising. It's all your body can handle right now. With that in mind:

→ Some of you will want to stick with your initial workout for the first week or three.

→ Others will include incremental additions in volume and intensity from week to week.

→ Still others, those with previous experience in running and some fitness base, might begin adding minutes and intensity from workout to workout.

There isn't a perfect rule to guide your decision-making on these increases. Dr. George Sheehan, our sport's late, great physician and philosopher, wrote, "We are all an experiment of one." What works for one of us won't work for all of us—or maybe for anyone else at all.

Especially in these first weeks, it pays to err on the side of caution. And with that in mind, two *imperfect* rules for you to consider are the "10 percent rule" and the "three-week rule."

The 10 percent rule recommends increasing your training volume by no more than 10 percent per week in order to avoid injures. For years, the 10 percent rule has been treated as the gold standard in running. Unfortunately, it's supported by anecdotal evidence, not science. In fact, a 2007 Dutch study following more than five hundred runners found identical injury rates for novice runners using the 10 percent rule and for those who increased their training more quickly. The 10 percent rule is also impractical. For example, if you start your program by walking ten minutes per day, it will take you over two months (using the 10 percent rule) to increase that amount to twenty minutes per day. Patience is one thing. Waiting through several reincarnations to build up to your first marathon is another.

I prefer the "three-week rule." With the three-week rule, you make very minor alterations in training volume from week to week, then schedule a larger increase in volume and intensity every three weeks. Three weeks usually gives your body adequate time to adjust to the bump in workload. If you need more than three weeks, you take it. The sample training schedules that appear at the end of Chapter 6 follow the three-week rule.

Deciding how many days per week to exercise

Most runners start their programs with three to four workouts per week. Runners with medical issues might opt for only two days at this stage. Runners who have running backgrounds or who have maintained fitness in other sports sometimes begin with more days. As a general guide:

→ **New runners:** 3–4 days per week

→ **Returning runners (no running for 3+ years):** 3–5 days per week

→ **Returning runners (some running past 3 years):** 3–6 days per week

→ **Current endurance background (trained in some other sport):** 3–7 days per week

Before you settle on the number of days you want to exercise, remember that you'll need to schedule adequate recovery. For runners without any background in the sport, even workouts that feel "easy" will register as "hard" for your body. That's because "hard" isn't defined by how you feel when exercising; it's determined by how long it takes your body to recover from the effort. If you haven't trained in the past (or haven't done any physical exercise in the recent past), then all workouts will require approximately two days of recovery (i.e., you can exercise every other day). For those runners who are more fit at the starts of their programs, you'll be able to schedule workouts on back-to-back days, but you'll also have to follow the hard-easy approach introduced in "Principle 6" (Chapter 2, page 20). If, after scheduling recovery days, you find you're still fatigued and sore for the next workout, add additional recovery days. Also, remember that it's essential to consume sufficient calories and log plentiful sleep (ideally seven to nine hours) during these first few weeks.

BECOMING A RUNNER: *Chuck Coats*

Chuck Coats, age fifty-six, started running in the sixth grade, set school records at Crook County High School (Prineville, Oregon), subsequently vanished from the running scene, and then, more than two decades later, reappeared to set an American age-group (forty-five to forty-nine) record for 3000 meters on the track. What occurred between high school and that American record, however, is mostly an alcoholic blur. "There's a lot of stuff I can't remember," says Chuck, "because I partied too hard." Chuck grew up on a farm, waking at 5 AM to feed the animals—the cows, chickens, pigs, and horses—and doing other farm chores, like hauling hay and chopping wood. It was hard work that prepared Chuck for his eventual career as a heavy highway construction laborer. After flunking out of college, he quit running, married his non-running sweetheart, Connie, and embarked on a life of work and partying. That lifestyle came to an abrupt halt in 1999, when the last in a line of DUIs provided a reality check. "It was either I get sober, or I'm going to sit in jail for a long time." Chuck stopped drinking, and he returned to running. "Those first six months were a living hell," he says. "My body couldn't do it." But he persevered, and running became his new addiction. "I'd work eight hours. Then go running. Then sleep. Then race every weekend." Along the way, Chuck developed into one of the top age-group runners in the United States. Then, in

Many runners resent the first few weeks of training. They feel hamstrung by the limited workouts. And by their lack of fitness. They dream of the day they can run for an hour straight without a break—and without the fatigue that cripples them after only a few minutes at the start of their programs.

Not me.

I've always loved the start of a running program.

I can't imagine anything better than the very first day.

January 2010, Connie became ill. "I took her into emergency," says Chuck, "and they found a lesion on one of her lungs." In March, she was diagnosed with lung cancer. Chuck took time off from work, and he and Connie went traveling. "The last six months of our life together was so powerful," says Chuck. "I fell in love all over again." Connie made Chuck promise to keep running, as a tool in his sobriety kit. And a few months after Connie passed, Chuck ran the California International Marathon in her honor. "When I finished the marathon," says Chuck, "I was in tears. I had some of Connie's ashes put into my necklace. So she was running right there with me. That's the first time she was ever able to go out running with me." Recently, Chuck traveled to the Coffee Creek Women's Correctional Institute to share his story with some inmates, then to take them on a short run. He loved it. They loved it. And he's scheduled to do it again. "How cool is that?" he says. "I spent some time in jail, because of my drinking. And to know they're getting it, to let them know that if this old drunk can go out and do it, then maybe they can, too. It's the neatest feeling."

That's because anything I do on day one, any workout at all, will lead to better fitness. If I walk around the block, I'll be a fitter runner tomorrow. If I throw in a few short surges of jogging, I might be fitter still. At no time, in the weeks and months and even years that I'll continue to work my running program, will I ever get as much fitness bang for my exercise buck as I will on that first day.

Or as you will on yours.

The only thing—the *only* thing—you'll need to watch out for is doing *too* much. Because if you overwhelm your body with an effort from which it can't recover, then guess what? It won't recover. So don't do that.

It takes courage to start a running program. But it takes exceptional courage to sign up for the patience, discipline, and perseverance that will be required to travel the road ahead.

CHAPTER TAKEAWAY

It's counterproductive to start a running program by mapping out a challenging training schedule. Your body isn't ready for that. Your muscles, bones, and tendons are too weak. Your nervous system hasn't learned how to supervise an efficient stride. Instead, you should focus on the act of running. You should patiently strengthen all the components of your running body. In choosing your workouts, you'll want to make sure that both the volume and intensity are manageable—or else you'll increase your chance of injury. And you'll need to resist the urge to increase that volume and intensity at more than an incremental rate. During these first weeks, it's wise to develop your listening skills, the ability to process sensory feedback from your body while exercising. Your reward will be a body that's physically and mentally ready for a challenging training program.

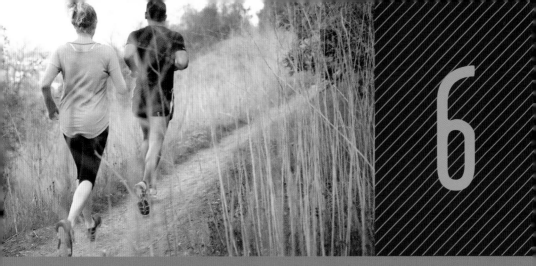

The Road Ahead

"Whether you think you can or think you can't, you're right."

—HENRY FORD

On my thirty-ninth birthday, for the first time in years, I laced up my running shoes and headed out the door for a planned thirty-minute jog. I managed to huff and puff for a torturous five minutes before exhaustion brought me to a standstill. I'd reached an intersection, the first stoplight on my route, and I remember thinking that if I rested just a little, bent over with my hands on my knees, eyeing the DON'T WALK signal, that maybe I'd recover by the time the signal changed to WALK. Instead, I felt worse. So I sat on the curb. And watched the signal blink back and forth from DON'T WALK to WALK to DON'T WALK to WALK until I wasn't even seeing it anymore, the sweat pouring off my forehead and stinging my eyes, my stomach cramping and my legs and arms all pins and needles, like they'd fallen asleep.

And I began to wonder if I'd be able to walk back home at all—or if maybe the cramping and numbness was going to work its way to somewhere more serious, like maybe to my heart. Which was all I needed. The anxiety on top of the exhaustion. But eventually my head began to clear. And my body began to recover. And I stood up and walked (slowly) back home.

My running goal after that day—and for months to come—was simple: Get healthy.

I wasn't training to run a marathon. Or to set age-group records. Or even to chase Zen bliss on long weekend runs through the local mountains.

My running goal was to *keep running*. It was to undo years of unhealthy behavior, of alcohol and tobacco and drug abuse. I didn't give a damn about my 5K time. I gave a damn about reclaiming my life, about waking up each morning feeling a little bit better than the previous morning. And so that's what I did. For more than a year.

As a result, I got healthier. And I got fitter. And I started thinking about running a race.

When the first race went well, I decided to run another.

Before you know it (OK, two or three years later), I'd switched from running to survive to running for competition, and then, a couple years after that, to running as part of my career, when I began writing for *Running Times* magazine and coaching professionally.

You have the power to choose your own running path. And, like me, you'll have the opportunity to amend that choice whenever and as often as you see fit.

This chapter will discuss a few paths that are available to you. And it will detail the types of training that accompany each. We'll also discuss exactly *how much* training—both distance running and high-intensity work—it takes to achieve improved fitness.

CHOOSING YOUR PATH

You have a vision of the runner you want to become. You had it when you got this book. And it's there still—if altered slightly by what you've read so far. The question now isn't whether you're ready to act on that vision. It's how best to achieve it.

First, you'll need to translate your vision into a more concrete goal. Yes, you want to run. But what's your endgame? Better health? Weight loss? Decreased stress? Increased happiness? A sense of accomplishment? A race? When you know your destination, it's easier to identify the path that will take you there. In this section, we'll look at five common running goals, along with an overview of the types of training required for each. We won't get into the specifics of the workouts mentioned (again, we'll define all of this book's workouts and learn how to perform them in Chapter 7), but you'll still get an idea of the training commitment that accompanies each goal. Of course, many (possibly most) of you won't fall neatly into these categories. And some of you are probably throwing your hands in the air right now and saying, "Whoa, I didn't sign up for this! I just want to run a few miles, a few times a week." I hear you, and we'll tackle the topic of a distance-only program right at the outset. Whatever your end goal, you should emerge from this chapter with a better sense of the workout load you're undertaking. And with a clearer vision of the road ahead.

Can I just run distance?

Yes, you can. You can train however you like. It's your running program. And an end goal is not a prerequisite to simply stepping out the door and putting in a couple/few miles at a time. The "12-Week Training Schedule for Beginning Runners" (page 110) will help launch you onto that path (just skip the slight increases in intensity that begin in week nine), or you can create a schedule of your own based upon the principles in this book. Many runners prefer the simplicity and familiarity of the same distance runs on the same days every week. If that's you, by all means travel that road.

But be aware that a distance-only program will limit the results you can expect to see from your running:

REDUCED FITNESS: You won't generate the same volume of fitness improvements as you could with a well-rounded schedule. You'll improve at a slower rate, and you'll limit your fitness potential. As a result, you'll feel more sluggish during your runs.

INJURY RISK: You'll be more susceptible to overuse and muscle-imbalance injuries. That's because you'll be training fewer muscle cells, using a reduced range of motion, and limiting your ability to rewire (improve) your nervous system.

LESS WEIGHT LOSS: You'll shed weight less quickly, since higher-intensity exercise is a key factor for increasing your metabolism when you're *not* exercising.

MUSCLE LOSS: At about age twenty-five, you begin to lose fast-twitch (speed and power) muscle cells at a rate of about 1 percent per year. The only way to arrest that loss is to train those cells—*intensely*. Distance runs train slow-twitch (endurance) muscle cells. So training only for distance won't save your faster muscle cells, and once they're gone, they're gone forever. When it comes to your muscles, a well-rounded program is one of nature's best strategies for fighting Father Time.

Again, there's no reason you can't limit your running to distance outings. But, if this is your plan, you should also ask yourself this question: "Why?" Maybe the various types of non-distance training sound too intimidating. Maybe you don't want to make that big of a commitment—you're tapped out just making the decision to run, *period*. Maybe you're afraid you won't be able to perform the exercises. Or that you might get injured trying them. Or something else.

Here's what I'd say in response: *Relax. Take a deep breath. Exhale.*

Remember that you'll have a few weeks of exercise under your belt before contemplating *any* workout (some very basic post-run exercises excluded) that isn't walking, jogging, or easy distance running. Even then, you won't be asked to tackle new exercises all at once. You'll take them one at a time, incorporating only the exercises you choose. And I promise you—*cross my heart*—that when the time comes, this training won't be nearly as intimidating as you think.

Let's imagine that you've never flown on a commercial airline before. And let's also imagine that I offered you a free plane ticket and a vacation to Hawaii. Sounds good, right? But then I start explaining the process of making your flight. First, you'd have to park off-site and take a shuttle to your airline. Then you'd wait in a check-in line—and probably have to manage the self-check-in kiosk. Your luggage would need to be limited to a certain size and weight. You could check some bags but keep others as carry-ons. You'd go through a security line, where you'd have to take off your shoes and other items of clothing, before stepping into a bomb-sniffing cubicle, raising your arms, and possibly being patted down by TSA agents. Next, you'd need to check for gate changes. Then line up to board the plane when your boarding group is called. And so on. My point is that catching a plane would probably sound pretty intimidating if you'd never done it before. But once you made it to your seat on the plane, you'd realize that it wasn't actually that bad. What's more, you'd be on a plane to Hawaii!

Scheduling workouts that go beyond simple distance runs is like that. With one important distinction: Once you start incorporating different workouts into your training, you'll discover that variety is, indeed, the spice of life; that's right, if you're like most runners, you'll actually enjoy the change of pace (literally) from day to day.

So, yes, you can run just distance. But a well-rounded program is the *best* way to improve performance, avoid injury, extend longevity, and keep running fun.

Training for general health

For both men and women, the desire to improve overall health is the number one motivation for running. If you're one of these runners, your goals include strengthening muscles, bones, and tendons; improving heart function and preventing heart disease; and reducing your odds of suffering from cancer, neurological problems, and age-related disabilities. If you're a parent, you might also be trying to improve your tag, chase, wrestling, and general playground stamina. Or maybe, for you, it's about creating base fitness for other activities: pickup basketball, weekend hikes, scuba diving, soccer, or virtually any sport on the planet.

YOUR PATH: If this is you, you can afford to go slowly with your program. You don't have to cram for a specific race date, a local Memorial Day 10K or a big-city marathon. And you're not frantic to drop fifty pounds for an upcoming event (e.g., your ten-year high school reunion or a wedding). Health is a lifelong goal. There's no rush. Your emphasis will be on creating a sustainable program that fits neatly into your non-running schedule. You'll want to make aerobic exercise (walking and distance running) the foundation of your program. And you'll probably want to expand on the Beginner's Body Strengthening routine (page 275), adding more exercises to your routine, as well as graduating to exercises with weights (e.g., handheld dumbbells). You'll need to train three to five times per week, depending on your initial fitness, non-running schedule, and motivation, and you won't need to progress to high-volume or high-intensity workouts.

RECOMMENDED WORKOUTS: walking, jogging, distance runs, resistance training, stretching

OPTIONAL WORKOUTS: strides, fartlek, cross training, balance

Training for weight loss

Weight loss is the second-most-popular motive for starting a running program. There's a reason for that. Running is the most effective exercise there is for shedding pounds (we'll discuss the reasons for this in Chapter 11, "Eat, Drink, and ~~Be Merry~~ Watch Your Calories"). While you've been patient until now, adhering to Chapter 2's Principle 9, "Dieting can wait" (page 23), you're ready to get back to your prime directive. You're ready to slim down.

YOUR PATH: First, you'll need to read this book's Chapter 11. It outlines your nutritional needs during a running program and explains the physiological process of losing weight. For training, you'll want to focus on distance runs, supplemented by sessions of resistance training (two to three times per week). Conversational distance runs (runs performed at a pace that allows you to easily manage conversation with a training partner) burn approximately 75 calories of fat per mile. If you run faster than that (e.g., repetitions and tempo efforts), you burn less fat and more carbohydrates, and you'll feel hungrier afterward—not the best recipe for weight loss. At the highest-intensity efforts, however, a funny thing happens: You slam the brakes on burning carbohydrates and get almost *all* of your energy from fat. So not only will the Beginner's Body Strengthening routine ward off injuries, it'll burn more fat; ditto for running sessions that include strides and fartlek. Both distance runs and resistance training have the added effect of keeping your metabolism elevated throughout the day. That means a higher daily calorie burn. The more days you exercise, the more weight you'll lose, so schedule at least three and up to seven days of training per week.

RECOMMENDED WORKOUTS: walking, jogging, distance runs, strides, resistance training, stretching

OPTIONAL WORKOUTS: long runs, fartlek, cross training, balance

Training as a hobby

Some of us just like to run, even if we can't quite put a finger on the reason why. Sure, we'd like to be healthier. Who wouldn't? And if a Sunday long run earns you an extra slice of pie, that's great, too. But if this is you, your reasons for running are probably a little more ethereal. Maybe you want to satisfy your nomadic spirit—to log expeditions into local mountains, along the beach, or through area parks. Maybe you want to feel the layers of stress peel away as you put life's daily grind behind you (or to rip them free with a music-driven, heart-pounding assault on the local roads and trails). Maybe you're looking to fortify your social experience by training with friends or a club, by turning every Saturday or Sunday morning into an adventure, into a shared journey in every physical, mental, and topographical sense. Or maybe you're not even sure what drives you. The thing is, at the risk of repeating myself, you just like to run.

YOUR PATH: If you're like the hobby runners I know, you aren't interested in the rigid discipline practiced by runners with health, weight, or race goals. You want to go with the flow, to run what you want when you want. If you decide to charge hard for three or four or ten miles, you want your body equipped for the effort. Ditto for a leisurely two-hour weekend excursion with your training group. You don't need a regimented progression of workouts. You need the fitness both to surge and to stroll. So you'll want to focus your training energy on two workouts: a weekly long run and a weekly repetition/tempo workout, supplemented by easy distance runs. The long runs will prepare you for those priceless weekend journeys. The faster-paced work will develop the strength, speed, and nervous system fine-tuning you need to charge. You'll require at least a couple of days a week for recovery from these outings, so plan on three to five runs per week.

RECOMMENDED WORKOUTS: walking, jogging, distance runs, long runs, repetitions, tempo, resistance training, stretching

OPTIONAL WORKOUTS: strides, fartlek, hill repeats, cross training, balance

Training for race completion

If your goal is to complete a race, you probably have a specific distance in mind. Maybe you want to run a 5K. Or a 10K. Of a half marathon or marathon. The thing is, your goal doesn't include running until your eyes bleed, then out-leaning some stranger at the finish line. That's not how you roll. For you, it's not about finish place. Or time. It's about going the distance. George Mallory, an early twentieth-century explorer, famously answered the question of why he wanted to climb Mount Everest with three words, "Because it's there." If you're training for race completion, you share the same mind-set. You want to claim your own mountain peak, represented by a race distance. For you, a race is something you can wrap your motivation around better than vague concepts like "fitness" and "health." Best of all, there'll be hundreds or even thousands of other runners in a race to share the experience with you.

YOUR PATH: You'll need to develop the necessary endurance to finish the race. For a 5K, this might require only a few weeks of training. For a marathon, you'll need at least a few months (even fit runners begin marathon training three to four months out from their goal race). While you'll need to incrementally increase the volume of all your runs, it's your weekly long run that's most important. You'll want to lengthen your long run until it's close to the length of your goal race. For a 5K, this means two to three miles. For a half marathon or marathon, you'll use minutes rather than miles as your yardstick, with your goal being to match in minutes your expected time for the race—the caveat being that a novice runner should never exceed a run of 2.5 hours, an experienced runner 3.5 hours. And, no, that won't be long enough to match most of your expected marathon finish times, but going longer than that invites injury and burnout. These long runs will prepare both your mind and body for the challenge of the race. Resistance training will also be an important part of your program, helping to offset muscle imbalances that might develop from an endurance-heavy schedule. Depending on your race goal, you might train as few as three days per week or as many as seven.

RECOMMENDED WORKOUTS: walking, jogging, distance runs, long runs (based upon race goal), resistance training, stretching

OPTIONAL WORKOUTS: strides, fartlek, repetitions, tempo, cross training, balance

Training to compete

Finally, we have the competitor. The competitor doesn't train to complete a race. He or she trains to own it. If this is you, you have two performance goals in mind. You want to beat other competitors. And you want to beat the clock. When the late Steve Prefontaine, known simply as "Pre" to his fans, said, "Somebody may beat me, but they are going to have to bleed to do it," you know exactly how he felt. It isn't that you don't feel a sense of accomplishment when you cross finish lines. It's just that racing other people and the clock, for you, is *fun.* Just as a gambler enjoys the rush of watching the roulette wheel spin, you live for the anxiety on the start line, the tension that mounts as you receive race splits (your elapsed time at specific spots on the course), and the physical and mental challenge of the long sprint to the finish.

YOUR PATH: The competitive runner has to train it all: distance runs, repetitions, tempo, drills, resistance training, cross training, and more. You'll need to increase both volume and intensity. Unlike training for race completion, your distance runs won't be based on goal race distance. Instead, you'll run as far (during both regular distance runs and your weekly long run) as it takes to create the optimum training stimulus. You'll include repetition workouts based on current and goal race effort. And speed work, such as fast track repetitions and hill sprints, at near-maximum effort. You'll incorporate as much resistance training, plyometrics, and drills as it takes to create the best stride possible. And you'll do all of this regardless of your goal race distance—because in the world of competitive distance running, there isn't a huge difference between the training of marathoners and 5K runners. Marathoners do a few longer runs, and 5K runners do a few more faster-paced repetition workouts. But 90 percent of the training is the same. For best results, you'll want to train four to seven days per week.

RECOMMENDED WORKOUTS: walking, jogging, distance runs, long runs, strides, fartlek, hill repeats, repetitions, tempo, speed work, resistance training, stretching

OPTIONAL WORKOUTS: downhill running, form drills, plyometrics, cross training, balance

SO JUST HOW MUCH RUNNING ARE WE TALKING ABOUT?

That's a good question. And the answer is: It's entirely up to you.

There is no universal prescription for running volume and training intensity. Not even for runners with the same running goal. Let's say your goal is to race a 5K. You can do that on as little as ninety minutes of training per week. But to run your best, you'll have to train three times that much. And an elite runner might log ten hours (or more) per week. What's more, the breakdown of that training can differ markedly. A runner looking to *complete* a 5K might only do aerobic running in the buildup to race day. A runner who wants to *compete* will have to set aside 15 to 20 percent of his or her training for higher-intensity efforts (repetitions, tempo, etc.).

You might also be coping with some obstacle that impacts your running. My history of smoking, drinking, and drugging made the first six months of my running program a real struggle. Runners with serious weight issues might have to schedule all walking and cross training in lieu of actual running until they've reached a predetermined goal weight (agreed upon with their physician or other health professional). And runners battling biomechanical and medical issues, such as asthma, chronic tendinitis, or amputation, will also require an individualized approach. And so on.

Top Reason Men Start Running (% of All Male Runners)

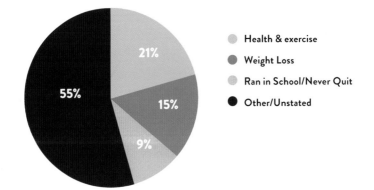

- Health & exercise
- Weight Loss
- Ran in School/Never Quit
- Other/Unstated

Top Reason Women Start Running (% of All Female Runners)

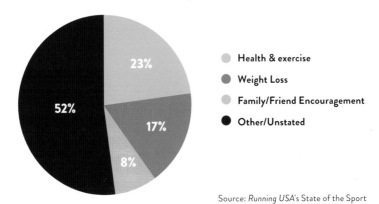

- Health & exercise
- Weight Loss
- Family/Friend Encouragement
- Other/Unstated

Source: *Running USA*'s State of the Sport

The truth is that there's no one-size-fits-all answer to the question: *How much?*

Luckily, for most of you, your first few months won't require major decision-making on this issue. That's because most running programs don't differ that much during the first few months. You're just trying to get your running legs under you. The incremental nature of training means that none of your potential paths will veer very far from any other, making course corrections or path substitutions easy to implement.

How fit is fit enough?

All running programs share the goal of improved fitness, which we'll define as the measure of our physical and mental health, as well as of our capacity for exercise. Regardless of whether you're training to ward off heart disease, lose weight, or run a 5K, you want to improve your fitness. Of course, different running paths have different goal fitness levels:

TRAINING FOR GENERAL HEALTH: See the recommendations from the American College of Sports Medicine (ACSM) below.

TRAINING FOR WEIGHT LOSS: You achieve and maintain your desired weight loss.

TRAINING FOR RACE COMPLETION: You finish your goal race (unless, of course, you decide you need to run another, possibly longer race).

TRAINING FOR COMPETITION: You set personal bests (PBs) in your goal race(s) and are satisfied that you can't get any faster.

If your fitness goal is less concrete than weight loss or running a race, you might want to consider the ACSM's recommended goals for a healthy fitness program:

→ Five days of 30–60 minutes of moderate-intensity exercise (e.g., walking or jogging) per week, *or* three days of 20–60 minutes of more vigorous exercise (e.g., faster running)

→ 2–3 days of resistance training per week

→ 2–3 days of flexibility exercises per week

→ 2–3 days of *neuromotor* exercise per week (i.e., balance, agility, and coordination)

Remember that those are *goals*. You build up to them. You don't start at that level. And if you follow the running programs in this book, including the Beginner's Body Strengthening routine, you'll eventually meet all those goals.

How long is long enough?

When most of us think about running, we think about distance. And when we think about distance, we think about the minutes (or miles) we'll be covering during our runs.

But exactly how far can you (or should you) run before the law of diminishing returns stops rewarding your effort? Your goal is to get fit. Not injured. Not bone-tired. Is thirty minutes enough? An hour? Two hours? More?

The answer is: It varies.

There are elite runners who train in excess of 150 miles per week; mind you, the ability (genetic and acquired) to train that far without breaking down is a big part of what makes them "elite." In contrast, many novice runners targeting their first 5K never exceed thirty minutes for a single run.

Your approach shouldn't be to emulate the volume of some other runner. It should be to learn, through experience, what volume is best for you. Here are some simple guidelines for increasing your mileage:

→ Increase your daily or weekly volume in small increments. At the outset of your program, increases of about 5–10 minutes per run every 2–3 weeks are manageable.

→ Make sure you're comfortable with your current volume before scheduling an increase.

→ Make your weekly long run 25–50 percent longer than your regular distance runs.

In the beginning, every walk or run you do will trigger major fitness adaptations. But as your fitness improves, it will take progressively larger increases in volume to trigger similar improvements (that *law of diminishing returns* we mentioned above). At that point, you'll have to weigh continued improvement against the rising risk of injury and physical burnout.

Most runners, at some point, settle on a weekly volume that satisfies their fitness goals without leaving themselves too exhausted to enjoy the achievement.

How hard is hard enough?

When we talk about hard training, we're usually referring to high-intensity exercise like repetitions, speed work, hill repeats, plyometrics, and resistance training. Yes, there are days when even a ten- or fifteen-minute jog will feel "hard," but we aren't talking about your subjective experience. We're talking about the demand that the workout makes on your body—specifically, how long it will take your body to recover from the workout.

Hard workouts (like those mentioned above) train a greater percentage of your muscle cells and increase the training stimulus for your nervous system, energy systems, bones, tendons, and the rest of your running body. In the right dose, that's a good thing. You'll end up with:

→ Stronger muscles, bones, tendons, ligaments, etc.

→ The ability to produce more energy

→ A more efficient nervous system

All of that will make you a more efficient runner. And that's a very good thing. Efficient runners have better "running economy"—the ability to run farther and faster using less energy (calories and oxygen). If you were a car, improved running economy would be equivalent to better gas mileage.

So how much hard work should you schedule? Most runners can meet their program goals with a single session of hard running each week—sessions should include *one* type of harder running (maybe two), not all of them. Runners who plan to compete in races, however, will want to schedule two sessions of harder running per week.

AEROBIC AND ANAEROBIC ENERGY

Before we exit this chapter, I want to spend a minute discussing a science-y subject that's at the core of your training as a runner: the difference between aerobic and anaerobic exercise. It's not important that you become an expert on the underlying science (there will *not* be a quiz at the end of the chapter). But for a couple reasons that we'll get to shortly, it's important that you understand the basic facts about each energy source.

So here goes.

Aerobic energy is produced within each muscle cell by hundreds (sometimes thousands) of microscopic structures called *mitochondria,* often referred to as the "powerhouses of the cell" because they provide more than 90 percent of the energy that you use each day. In order to create all this energy, your "powerhouses" need two things: fuel and oxygen. They get the fuel (carbohydrates and fat) by breaking down the food you eat. The oxygen is delivered by your heart and blood vessels. When you exercise, you use a *lot* of aerobic energy. For a distance run, more than 99 percent of the energy you use will be aerobic energy. As you pick up the pace and shorten your running distance, the overall contribution of aerobic energy decreases. For a 5K race, it's still about 90 percent. If you race a mile, it drops to 75 percent. At very high running intensities (races of 400 meters or less), anaerobic energy becomes your main power source.

Anaerobic energy is produced within your muscle cells, too, but it's created without oxygen. You have two different sources of anaerobic energy. One provides a burst of high-octane energy that lasts a maximum of fifteen seconds—think the nitro boost by Dominic Toretto to rocket his RX-7 to victory in *The Fast and the Furious.* This is the energy source exploited by Usain Bolt and other sprinters when running the 100-meter dash. A second anaerobic source ramps up more slowly (but still one hundred times faster than aerobic energy production) and provides another minute of maximum-capacity energy production. The problem with this second source, however, is that the more of it you use, the more fatigued you become. Run all-out for a minute straight—draining this source—and your muscles will burn, your legs will turn to cement, and your pace will slow to a crawl (what 400- and 800-meter runners refer to as "booty lock"). What's more, it might take you a few days to recover from the effort.

To recap:

→ **Aerobic energy:** Requires oxygen and lasts long-term

→ **Anaerobic energy:** Doesn't require oxygen, is produced more quickly than aerobic energy, and is short-lived at maximum production (it can last longer at reduced production)

So why is the difference between aerobic and anaerobic energy important to you? I'm glad you asked. There are two main reasons it's important:

1 **AEROBIC ENERGY START-UP TIME:** When you start a run, it takes thirty to forty-five seconds to deliver increased amounts of oxygen to your muscles (via your lungs, heart, and blood), which means it takes thirty to forty-five seconds before your aerobic system can produce an increased energy supply (since it requires more oxygen to do so). Until that oxygen arrives, you have to rely on *anaerobic energy* to temporarily provide the extra energy that your body needs in order to exercise (i.e., to run). This is why the most anaerobic part of any run is the *first part*. This reliance on anaerobic energy will continue until your aerobic system can get up to speed—until your muscle cells receive the oxygen they need to produce enough aerobic energy to take over your energy needs. Because of this, you'll need to begin *each and every* workout with a short warm-up. When you start slowly—and, yes, some of the top runners in the world begin their distance runs by walking—you give your aerobic system a chance to keep pace with your energy requirements. You don't flood your system with anaerobic energy production, and you don't become overwhelmed by the fatigue that can accompany that production. You'll feel better. You'll run longer. And your body will thank you with faster recovery and greater improvement.

2 **ANAEROBIC TRAINING FOR RACING:** Those of you with race goals will need to train your bodies for the inevitable demand put on your anaerobic system at the beginning of a race, during the race

(as your body copes with the fatigue associated with anaerobic energy production), and at the end of the race, when your "kick" to the finish reengages your anaerobic energy production at full force. This will require that you incorporate anaerobic training into your program (e.g., Chapter 7's hill repeats, repetitions, and other speed work).

Beyond those two practical reasons for understanding your body's energy production, it's just kind of cool to know how you're fueling your workouts—and to recognize that your training will be vastly increasing your ability to produce *both* types of energy. If your energy source today is a pair of AAA batteries, it's about to become a bona fide industrial power station.

The best part of training is that the more you do it, the easier it gets. You get fitter. And then you get more fit still. And, finally, you achieve your running goal. That's the promise of a properly constructed training program. And that's what you can expect.

The only caveat I want to introduce, and please take this the way it's intended: You have to begin with a realistic and achievable plan. It breaks my heart when runners confess goals that are beyond their current grasp—not only because they'll fail to achieve the goal in the desired time frame, but because they'll miss the joy and sense of accomplishment that could be theirs by targeting milepost goals along the way. There's almost nothing you can't accomplish as a runner. But there are a whole slew of things that you can't accomplish in your first three months.

"Honesty is the first chapter in the book of wisdom," wrote Thomas Jefferson, in a letter to Nathaniel Macon, back in 1819. And, if Jefferson will allow us, it's also the first chapter in the book of running.

Start by being honest about your current fitness. I wanted to run thirty minutes on day one, but I could barely manage five. I readjusted, and because of that, I was able to train successfully—a program that continues strong fifteen years later.

Next, be honest about your initial running goal. On day one, I assumed I was ready to run. I wasn't. On day two, I adjusted my goal to basic fitness (a goal that was within reach) and changed my workout to a combination of walking and jogging. Later, I built upon successful completion of that goal, and, eventually, I ran better than I'd ever thought possible—and with the right approach, you can, too!

Finally, be honest about the obstacles you face. Yes, there is almost no obstacle you can't overcome, as the profiles in this book illustrate. But "overcome" is the key word. My smoking didn't vanish the first day I ran. Neither did my drinking. Or the drugs. Running doesn't make obstacles

BECOMING A RUNNER: *Greg Schnoor*

Greg Schnoor, age thirty-eight, of Pensacola, Florida, had sinus issues in his early thirties. He'd even had surgery for them. When the issues returned in 2010, he got a CT scan. "I knew something wasn't right when my doctor called me early the next morning," says Greg. "He told me there was a golf ball–sized area of swelling in my brain." An MRI confirmed the worst. Greg had a brain tumor. So on October 10, 2010, Greg had surgery. Then he got more bad news: Tests confirmed he'd had a grade 3 malignant brain tumor (an oligodendroglioma). He'd need six more weeks of radiation and chemotherapy—to be administered in Gainesville, in North Central Florida—to reduce the chance of recurrence. Greg's wife, Lisa, accompanied him to Gainesville, leaving their four children—sons Justin, Tony, and Riley, and two-month-old daughter Aloy—in Pensacola. "We'd just had our baby daughter," says Greg, "and now we had to leave her for six weeks. It was tough, dealing with that." Greg lost weight during the treatment, then promptly gained it back and more when he returned to Pensacola. "I thought, *What the hell am I doing to myself?* That's when I decided to start respecting my body. And that's when I started running." At first, he'd tag along on runs with his two older sons, who belonged to a youth running club. He began by running a mile. Then a couple of miles. Eventually, he entered his first 5K, at Universal Studios in Florida, where his family was vacationing on a trip paid for by Memories of Love—an organization that disappear. But smart, sustainable training will help you to overcome or circumvent them. We'll revisit this issue in Chapter 9, with the creation of your personal action plan.

The road ahead is long, and the journey will be challenging. But with honesty, patience, and perseverance, coupled with a good training plan, that isn't a bad thing.

Instead, it's what makes the road worth traveling.

provides memory-generating experiences for families with a parent who has a life-threatening illness. "I completed [the 5K], only stopping once or twice," says Greg. After that, he ran more often, and he began to add a mile every week to his Saturday long run. Still receiving chemo one week out of every month, Greg found that running improved his energy. "Chemo can really affect your body," he says. "I'd be just glued to the bed, not wanting to get up. It was hard to open my eyes." But with running, things changed. "I was doing 20-mile long runs during the weeks I got chemo." When Greg looked for a race that benefited brain cancer research, he couldn't find one nearby. "So I decided to start my own," he says. Drawing upon his skill as a web designer and online marketing consultant, he created the Brain Tumor Run for Research 5K, raising twenty thousand dollars after expenses the first year. Greg has now completed a half dozen marathons and three ultras, with more to come. "I'm not letting cancer plan my life," he says. "I almost feel like the cancer's got to catch me."

CHAPTER TAKEAWAY

To create a training program that's right for you, you must pick a running goal. This could be as simple as general health. Or weight loss. Or even running a race. Naturally, you can change goals at any time—or commit to a new goal once the current one is achieved. Once you know your goal, you'll be able to schedule the types of training that best suit that goal. All runners will want to build basic fitness. But beyond that, the volume of endurance training and harder work that you do will depend on your goal and your personal capacity (both mental and physical). Once you've decided on the correct training path for *you*, all that's left is to run it.

TRAINING SCHEDULES

THE FOLLOWING SAMPLE TRAINING SCHEDULES are meant to be used as guides for your own running program. Remember that each of us develops fitness at a unique rate, and you'll want to listen carefully to your body as you embark on any training schedule—and then make adjustments to your schedule as required (using what you've learned in this book to make informed decisions).

The schedules beginning on page 110 (all of which are available in easy-to-print format at bornagainrunner.com) include the following:

→ **12-Week Training Schedule for Beginning Runners (Noncompetitive):** This schedule is for new runners who want to run—period. You'll get your running legs under you, and you can always switch to a race-oriented schedule if your running goals change. *Page 110*

→ **12-Week Training Schedule for Beginning Runners (Competitive):** This schedule is for new runners who have the racing jones. The program is slightly accelerated and includes higher-intensity workouts than those in the noncompetitive schedule. *Page 111*

→ **12-Week Training Schedule for Returning Runners (Noncompetitive):** If you're returning to running after a brief break (say, under a year), this schedule offers an accelerated return to your previous form. *Page 112*

→ **12-Week Training Schedule for Returning Runners (Competitive):** Like the previous schedule, this one is for runners who've trained in the recent past. You'll increase your volume and intensity more quickly than with a new runner's schedule, and you'll be ready to race in twelve weeks. *Page 113*

→ **12-Week Training Schedule for Running (Next Phase) – Noncompetitive:** This schedule picks up where the "Beginning Runners (Noncompetitive)" schedule leaves off. *Page 114*

→ **12-Week Training Schedule for Competitive Running (Next Phase) – Multiple Schedules:** These two schedules pick up where the "Beginning Runners (Competitive)" schedule leaves off. There are schedules for three to four days and five to seven days of training per week. You'll be able to race at any time during these schedules using the "2-Week Training Adjustment for 5K or 10K Race" or the "3-Week Training Adjustment for Half Marathon Race" (page 117), after which you can return to the schedules exactly where you left off. The schedules will prepare you for any race from 5K to the Half Marathon. *Pages 115–17*

Most of the schedules include workouts that are to be completed at specific paces. For example, you might be asked to run "fast tempo" repetitions on the road or track intervals at "10K pace." As new and returning runners, you might not be clear on what's expected—time-wise or effort-wise—at each pace. Don't worry; there are two ways you can go:

1 **"COMPARABLE PERFORMANCE AND WORKOUT PACES TABLE" AT BORNAGAINRUNNER.COM:** If you know what your current 5K race time is (or can guesstimate within thirty seconds or so), you can use this table to find your training paces (and predicted race times for the 10K, half marathon, and marathon). Simply look up your 5K time (or the time that's closest to it) in the left-hand column of this table; all your training paces (from your distance runs to your 5K-paced repetitions) will be listed in that row. There's also an automated current and goal training pace calculator on the site; you'll just need to enter current and goal 5K times.

2 **GUESSTIMATE YOUR PACES:** Honestly, it's not about the pace. It's about the effort. Certain good things happen to your body when you train at different efforts. So until you race a 5K and collect a "current 5K time," you can base your effort for different workouts on the following easy breakdown:

→ **Slow Tempo:** You'll run slightly faster than conversational distance pace

→ **Fast Tempo:** Your breathing will pick up noticeably, but not so much that you're uncomfortable

→ **10K Pace:** Your breathing is definitely getting harder, and conversation isn't really an option

→ **5K Pace:** Now you're really breathing, and you'll start to feel fairly uncomfortable after 3–4 minutes—although you could keep up the pace for 15–20 minutes (yes, most of you will keep up the pace for longer in a race, but it's always much harder in a workout)

→ **Sub-5K Pace:** This is a pace that you could only sustain for 1–2 miles all-out

→ **Rule of Repetitions:** If all else fails, follow the rule of repetitions; in a repetitions workout, never run so hard that you couldn't add at least one more repetition at the end of the workout if required. In other words, pick a pace that you can handle and that won't destroy you.

Finally, you need to know how long each of your distance runs should last. Many of you will increase your runs incrementally until you find a run length that is right for you. But for those who need a hand in the process, I provide a "Length of Regular and Long Distance Runs" table at bornagainrunner.com. This table gives you an estimated length for both your regular distance runs and long runs based on the combination of your current 5K time and weekly mileage—yes, I know we've made a big point about not worrying so much about mileage, but for the sake of getting you this information in an easy-to-digest format, we'll make an exception in this case.

Good luck!

12-WEEK TRAINING SCHEDULE
FOR BEGINNING RUNNERS (NONCOMPETITIVE)

WEEK	SUN	MON	TUES	WED	THU	FRI	SAT
1	OFF	Easy Walking: 10–15 minutes	OFF	Easy Walking: 10–15 minutes	OFF	Easy Walking: 10–15 minutes	OFF or Easy Walking: 10–15 minutes
2	OFF	Easy Walking: 20 minutes	OFF	Brisk Walking: 15 minutes	OFF	Easy Walking: 20 minutes	OFF or Easy Walking: 10–15 minutes
3	OFF	Brisk Walking: 15–20 minutes	OFF	Easy Walking: 20 minutes	OFF	Walk/Jog: 15–20 minutes*	OFF or Easy Walking: 20 minutes
4	OFF	Walk/Jog: 20 minutes	OFF	Easy Walking: 20 minutes	OFF	Walk/Jog: 20 minutes	OFF or Easy Walking: 20 minutes or Cross Train
5	OFF	Walk/Jog: 20 minutes	OFF	Easy Walking: 20 minutes	OFF	Walk/Jog: 20 minutes	OFF or Easy Walking: 20 minutes or Cross Train
6	OFF	Walk/Jog: 20 minutes	OFF	Easy Walking: 20 minutes	OFF	Easy Distance Run: 20 minutes	OFF or Easy Walking: 20 minutes or Cross Train
7	OFF	Easy Distance Run: 20–30 minutes	OFF	Walk/Jog: 20–30 minutes	OFF	Easy Distance Run: 20–30 minutes	OFF or Walk/Jog: 20–30 minutes or Cross Train
8	OFF	Easy Distance Run: 20–30 minutes	OFF	Walk/Jog: 20–30 minutes	OFF	Easy Distance Run: 20–30 minutes	OFF or Walk/Jog: 20–30 minutes or Cross Train
9	OFF	Easy Distance Run: 20–30 minutes + 4 x Strides (60–80 meters)	OFF	Easy Distance Run: 20–25 minutes	OFF	Distance Run: 20–30 minutes	OFF or Walk/Jog: 20–30 minutes or Cross Train
10	OFF	Beginner's Fartlek: 15–20 minutes	OFF	Easy Distance Run: 20–30 minutes	OFF	Distance Run: 20–30 minutes	OFF or Easy Distance Run: 20–30 minutes or Cross Train
11	OFF	Long Run: 30–40 minutes + 6 x Strides (60–80 minutes)	OFF	Easy Distance Run: 20–30 minutes	OFF	Distance Run: 20–30 minutes	OFF or Easy Distance Run: 20–30 minutes or Cross Train
12	OFF	Beginner's Fartlek: 15–20 minutes	OFF	Easy Distance Run: 20–30 minutes	OFF	Distance Run: 20–40 minutes	OFF or Easy Distance Run: 20–30 minutes or Cross Train

* For Walk/Jog workouts, begin with jogging surges that match your fitness. That might mean 10–15 seconds for less-fit runners, and 1- to 3-minute surges for runners who are already fit from other activities. Gradually increase the length of your surges from week to week, and always walk for *at least* an equivalent time.

12-WEEK TRAINING SCHEDULE
FOR BEGINNING RUNNERS (COMPETITIVE)

WEEK	SUN	MON	TUES	WED	THU	FRI	SAT
1	OFF	Easy Walking: 10–15 minutes	OFF	Easy Walking: 10–15 minutes	OFF	Easy Walking: 10–15 minutes	OFF or Easy Walking: 10–15 minutes
2	OFF	Easy Walking: 20 minutes	OFF	Brisk Walking: 15 minutes	OFF	Walk/Jog: 20 minutes*	OFF or Easy Walking: 20 minutes
3	OFF	Walk/Jog: 20 minutes	OFF	Walk/Jog: 20 minutes	OFF	Easy Distance Run: 15–20 minutes	OFF or Easy Walking: 20–30 minutes
4	OFF	Easy Distance Run: 20 minutes + Strides	OFF	Easy Distance Run: 20 minutes	OFF	Walk/Jog: 20 minutes	Easy Distance Run: 20–30 minutes
5	OFF	Easy Distance Run: 20 minutes + Strides	OFF	Easy Distance Run: 20 minutes	OFF	Walk/Jog: 20 minutes	Easy Distance Run: 20–30 minutes
6	OFF	Easy Distance Run: 20 minutes + Strides	OFF	Easy Distance Run: 20 minutes	OFF	Easy Distance Run: 20 minutes	Distance Run: 30 minutes
7	OFF	Beginner's Fartlek: 10–25 minutes	OFF or Cross Train	Easy Distance Run: 20–30 minutes	OFF	Easy Distance Run: 20 minutes	Distance Run: 40 minutes
8	OFF	Fast Tempo-Pace Reps: 6 x 1 minute, with 2-minute jog between reps	OFF or Cross Train	Easy Distance Run: 20–30 minutes	OFF	Easy Distance Run: 20 minutes	Distance Run: 40 minutes
9	OFF	10K-Pace Reps: 5 x 2 minutes, with 3-minute jog between reps	OFF or Cross Train	Distance Run: 20–30 minutes	OFF	Easy Distance Run: 20 minutes	Long Run: 45–50 minutes
Continue with next three weeks, or join one of the "Running—Next Phase" programs (3-4, 5, 6, and 7 days per week), beginning with week 1							
10	OFF	10K-Pace Reps: 5 x 3 minutes, with 3-minute jog between reps	OFF or Cross Train	Distance Run: 20–40 minutes	Hill Strides: 15–20 seconds, with walk back to start line	OFF or Easy Distance Run: 20–40 minutes	Long Run: 45–50 minutes
11	OFF	Slow Tempo-Pace Reps: 3 x 5 minutes, with 3-minute jog between reps	OFF or Cross Train	Distance Run: 20–40 minutes	Hill Repeats: 8 x 30 seconds, with 90-second jog/walk between reps	OFF or Easy Distance Run: 20–40 minutes	Long Run: 45–50 minutes
12	OFF	5K-Pace Reps: 4 x 3 minutes, with 3-minute jog between reps	OFF or Cross Train	Distance Run: 20–40 minutes	Distance Run: 20 minutes, with 4 x strides at end of run (5K effort)	OFF or Easy Distance Run: 20 minutes	5K RACE

* For Walk/Jog workouts, begin with jogging surges that match your fitness. That might mean 10–15 seconds for less-fit runners, and 1- to 3-minute surges for runners who are already fit from other activities. Gradually increase the length of your surges from week to week, and always walk for *at least* an equivalent time.

12-WEEK TRAINING SCHEDULE
FOR RETURNING RUNNERS (NONCOMPETITIVE)

WEEK	SUN	MON	TUES	WED	THU	FRI	SAT
1 Base Training	OFF	Easy Walking: 10–15 minutes	OFF	Easy Walking: 10–15 minutes	OFF	Optional Cross Training Day: 10–15 minutes	Easy Walking: 10–15 minutes
2 Base Training	OFF	Easy Walking: 30 minutes	OFF	Walk/Jog: 20–30 minutes; include 10 x 30-second jog-surges (at least 1 minute between)	OFF	Optional Cross Training Day: 10–15 minutes	Walk/Jog: 30–45 minutes; include 10 x 30-second jog-surges (at least 1 minute recovery)
3 Base Training	OFF	Walk/Run: 30 minutes—alternate 1-minute run with 1-minute walk	OFF	Distance Run: 2 x 10 minutes, with 3-minute walk between reps	OFF	Optional Cross Training Day: 15–20 minutes	Distance Run: 2 x 10 minutes, with 3-minute walk between reps
1	OFF	Regular Distance: 20–25 minutes	OFF	Regular Distance: 20–25 minutes	OFF	Optional Cross Training Day: 20–25 minutes	Regular Distance: 20–25 minutes + 4 x strides (60–80 meters)
2	OFF	Fast Tempo-Pace Reps: 6 x 1 minute, with 2-minute jog between reps	OFF	Regular Distance: 20–25 minutes + 4 strides (during last 5 minutes of run or post-run)	OFF	Optional Cross Training Day: 20–25 minutes	Regular Distance: 20–25 minutes
3	OFF	Beginner's Fartlek: 15–20 minutes	OFF	Regular Distance: 25–30 minutes + 4 strides (during last 5 minutes of run or post-run)	OFF	Optional Cross Training Day: 25–30 minutes	Long Run: 30–40 minutes
4	OFF	Slow Tempo-Pace Reps: 6 x 2 minutes, with 3-minute jog between reps	Optional Distance Run or Cross Training Day: 25–30 minutes	Regular Distance: 25–30 minutes + 4 strides (during last 5 minutes of run or post-run)	OFF	Optional Distance Run or Cross Training Day: 25–30 minutes	Long Run: 30–40 minutes
5	OFF	Beginner's Fartlek: 15–20 minutes	Optional Distance Run or Cross Training Day: 30–40 minutes	Regular Distance: 30–40 minutes + 4 strides (during last 5 minutes of run or post-run)	OFF	Optional Distance Run or Cross Training Day: 30–40 minutes	Long Run: 45–50 minutes
6	OFF	Fast Tempo-Pace Reps: 4 x 3 minutes, with 3-minute jog between reps	Optional Distance Run or Cross Training Day: 30–40 minutes	Regular Distance: 30–40 minutes + 4 strides (during last 5 minutes of run or post-run)	OFF	Optional Distance Run or Cross Training Day: 30–40 minutes	Long Run: 45–50 minutes
Continue with final six weeks, or join the "Running—Next Phase (Noncompetitive)" program beginning with week 3 or 4							
7	OFF	Hill Repeats: 8 x 20 seconds, with 60-second jog/walk between reps	Optional Distance Run or Cross Training Day: 30–40 minutes	Regular Distances: 30–40 minutes + 4–6 strides (during last 5 minutes of run or post-run)	OFF	Optional Distance Run or Cross Training Day: 30–40 minutes	Long Run: 45–50 minutes
8	OFF	10K-Pace Reps: 6 x 2 minutes, with 3-minute jog between reps	Optional Distance Run or Cross Training Day: 45–50 minutes	Regular Distance: 45–50 minutes + 4–6 strides (during last 5 minutes of run or post-run)	OFF	Optional Distance Run or Cross Training Day: 45–50 minutes	Long Run: 60–65 minutes
9	OFF	Hill Repeats: 8 x 30 seconds, with 90-second jog/walk between reps	Optional Distance Run or Cross Training Day: 45–50 minutes	Regular Distance: 45–50 minutes + 4–6 strides (during last 5 minutes of run or post-run)	OFF	Optional Distance Run or Cross Training Day: 45–50 minutes	Long Run: 60–65 minutes
10	OFF	Fast Tempo-Pace Reps: 4 x 5 minutes, with 3-minute jog between reps	Optional Distance Run or Cross Training Day: 45–50 minutes	Regular Distance: 45–50 minutes + 4–6 strides (during last 5 minutes of run or post-run)	OFF	Optional Distance Run or Cross Training Day: 45–50 minutes	Long Run: 60–65 minutes
11	OFF	Hill Repeats: 8 x 30 seconds, with 90-second jog/walk between reps	Optional Distance Run or Cross Training Day: 55–60 minutes	Regular Distance: 55–60 minutes + 4–6 strides (during last 5 minutes of run or post-run)	OFF	Optional Distance Run or Cross Training Day: 55–60 minutes	Long Run: 70–80 minutes (or stay at 60–65 minutes—your choice)
12	OFF	10K-Pace Reps: 4 x 3 minutes, with 3-minute jog between reps	Optional Distance Run or Cross Training Day: 55–60 minutes	Regular Distance: 55–60 minutes + 4–6 strides (during last 5 minutes of run or post-run)	OFF	Optional Distance Run or Cross Training Day: 55–60 minutes	Long Run: 70–80 minutes (or stay at 60–65 minutes—your choice)

12-WEEK TRAINING SCHEDULE
FOR RETURNING RUNNERS (COMPETITIVE)

WEEK	SUN	MON	TUES	WED	THU	FRI	SAT
1 *Base Training*	OFF	Easy Walking: 10–15 minutes	OFF	Easy Walking: 10–15 minutes	OFF	Optional Cross Training Day: 10–15 minutes	Easy Walking: 10–15 minutes
2 *Base Training*	OFF	Easy Walking: 30 minutes	OFF	Walk/Jog: 20–30 minutes; include 10 x 30-second jog-surges (at least 1 minute between surges)	OFF	Optional Cross Training Day: 10–15 minutes	Walk/Jog: 30–45 minutes; include 10 x 30-second jog-surges (at least 1 minute recovery)
3 *Base Training*	OFF	Walk/Run: 30 minutes— alternate 1-minute run with 1-minute walk	OFF	Distance Run: 2 x 10 minutes, with 3-minute walk between reps	OFF	Optional Cross Training Day: 15–20 minutes	Distance Run: 2 x 10 minutes, with 3-minute walk between reps
1	OFF	Regular Distance: 20–25 minutes	OFF	Regular Distance: 20–25 minutes	OFF	Optional Cross Training Day: 20–25 minutes	Distance Run: 20–25 minutes; include 10 x 20-second surges at 10K effort, with 40-second jog between reps
2	OFF	Fast Tempo-Pace Reps: 6 x 1 minute, with 2-minute jog between reps	OFF	Regular Distance: 20–25 minutes	OFF	Optional Cross Training Day: 20–25 minutes	Regular Distance: 20–25 minutes
3	OFF	10K-Pace Reps: 5 x 2 minutes, with 3-minute jog between reps	OFF	Regular Distance: 20–25 minutes	OFF	Optional Cross Training Day: 25–30 minutes	Long Run: 30–40 minutes
4	OFF	Slow Tempo-Pace Reps: 3 x 5 minutes, with 3-minute jog between reps	Optional Distance Run or Cross Training Day: 25–30 minutes	Regular Distance: 20–25 minutes	OFF	Optional Distance Run or Cross Training Day: 25–30 minutes	Long Run: 30–40 minutes
5	OFF	5K-Pace Reps: 4 x 3 minutes, with 3-minute jog between reps	Optional Distance Run or Cross Training Day: 30–40 minutes	Hill Repeats: 8 x 30 seconds, with 60-second jog/walk between reps	OFF	Optional Distance Run or Cross Training Day: 30–40 minutes	Long Run: 45–50 minutes
6	OFF	Slow Tempo-Pace Reps: 2 x 10 minutes, with 3-minute jog between reps	Optional Distance Run or Cross Training Day: 30–40 minutes	Hill Repeats: 4 x 60 seconds, with 3-minute jog/walk between reps	OFF	Optional Distance Run or Cross Training Day: 30–40 minutes	Long Run: 45–50 minutes
Continue with final six weeks, or join one of the "Running—Next Phase" programs (3–4, 5, 6, and 7 days per week), beginning with week 3 or 4							
7	OFF	10K-Pace Reps: 4 x 4 minutes, with 3-minute jog between reps	Optional Distance Run or Cross Training Day: 30–40 minutes	Road Intervals: 10 x 30 seconds (sub-5K effort), with 60-second jog between reps	OFF	Optional Distance Run or Cross Training Day: 30–40 minutes	Long Run: 35–40 minutes (scaled back for 1 week as part of scheduled recovery)
8	OFF	Fast Tempo-Pace Reps: 4 x 5 minutes, with 3-minute jog between reps	Optional Distance Run or Cross Training Day: 45–50 minutes	Hill Repeats: 6 x 60 seconds, with 3-minute jog/walk between reps	OFF	Optional Distance Run or Cross Training Day: 45–50 minutes	Long Run: 60–65 minutes
9	OFF	5K-Pace Reps: 4 x 4 minutes, with 3-minute jog between reps	Optional Distance Run or Cross Training Day: 45–50 minutes	Hill Repeats: 4 x 90 seconds, with 5-minute jog/walk between reps	OFF	Optional Distance Run or Cross Training Day: 45–50 minutes	Long Run: 60–65 minutes
10	OFF	Fast Tempo-Pace Reps: 2 x 10 minutes, with 3-minute jog between reps	Optional Distance Run or Cross Training Day: 45–50 minutes	Road Intervals: 15 x 30 seconds (sub-5K effort), with 60-second jog between reps	OFF	Optional Distance Run or Cross Training Day: 45–50 minutes	Long Run: 60–65 minutes
11	OFF	10K-Pace Reps: 4 x 5 minutes, with 3-minute jog between reps	Optional Distance Run or Cross Training Day: 55–60 minutes	Hill Repeats: 4 x 90 seconds, with 5-minute jog/walk between reps	OFF	Optional Distance Run or Cross Training Day: 55–60 minutes	Long Run: 70–80 minutes
12	Race Week: Use the "2-Week Training Adjustment for 5K or 10K Race" (page 117) to prepare for your first race						RACE

12-WEEK TRAINING SCHEDULE
FOR RUNNING (NEXT PHASE) - NONCOMPETITIVE

WEEK	SUN	MON	TUES	WED	THU	FRI	SAT
1	OFF	Fast Tempo-Pace Reps: 4 x 5 minutes, with 3-minute jog between reps	Your option: Distance Run, Cross Training, or OFF	Distance Run	Your option: Distance Run, Cross Training or OFF	Your option: Distance Run, Cross Training, or OFF	Long Run
2	OFF	Hill Repeats: 8 x 20 seconds, with 60-second jog/walk between reps	Your option: Distance Run, Cross Training, or OFF	Distance Run	Your option: Distance Run, Cross Training, or OFF	Your option: Distance Run, Cross Training, or OFF	Long Run
3	OFF	10K-Pace Reps: 8 x 1 minute, with 2-minute jog between reps	Your option: Distance Run, Cross Training, or OFF	Distance Run	Your option: Distance Run, Cross Training, or OFF	Your option: Distance Run, Cross Training, or OFF	Long Run
4	OFF	Fast Tempo-Pace Reps: 2 x 10 minutes, with 3-minute jog between reps	Your option: Distance Run, Cross Training, or OFF	Distance Run	Your option: Distance Run, Cross Training, or OFF	Your option: Distance Run, Cross Training, or OFF	Long Run
5	OFF	Hill Repeats: 8 x 30 seconds, with 90-second jog/walk between reps	Your option: Distance Run, Cross Training, or OFF	Distance Run	Your option: Distance Run, Cross Training, or OFF	Your option: Distance Run, Cross Training, or OFF	Long Run
6	OFF	10K-Pace Reps: 6 x 2 minutes, with 3-minute jog between reps	Your option: Distance Run, Cross Training, or OFF	Distance Run	Your option: Distance Run, Cross Training, or OFF	Your option: Distance Run, Cross Training, or OFF	Long Run
7	OFF	Fast Tempo: 15–20 minutes	Your option: Distance Run, Cross Training, or OFF	Distance Run	Your option: Distance Run, Cross Training, or OFF	Your option: Distance Run, Cross Training, or OFF	Long Run
8	OFF	Hill Repeats: 6 x 45 seconds, with 3-minute jog/walk between reps	Your option: Distance Run, Cross Training, or OFF	Distance Run	Your option: Distance Run, Cross Training, or OFF	Your option: Distance Run, Cross Training, or OFF	Long Run
9	OFF	10K-Pace Reps: 4 x 3 minutes, with 3-minute jog between reps	Your option: Distance Run, Cross Training, or OFF	Distance Run	Your option: Distance Run, Cross Training, or OFF	Your option: Distance Run, Cross Training, or OFF	Long Run
10	OFF	Slow Tempo: 20–30 minutes	Your option: Distance Run, Cross Training, or OFF	Distance Run	Your option: Distance Run, Cross Training, or OFF	Your option: Distance Run, Cross Training, or OFF	Long Run
11	OFF	Hill Repeats: 6 x 60 seconds, with 4-minute jog/walk between reps	Your option: Distance Run, Cross Training, or OFF	Distance Run	Your option: Distance Run, Cross Training, or OFF	Your option: Distance Run, Cross Training, or OFF	Long Run
12	OFF	10K-Pace Reps: 4 x 3 minutes, with 3-minute jog between reps	Your option: Distance Run, Cross Training, or OFF	Distance Run	Your option: Distance Run, Cross Training, or OFF	Your option: Distance Run, Cross Training, or OFF	Long Run

Continued Training: If you decide to remain noncompetitive, you can recycle your last six weeks of this program to maintain fitness; you can increase or decrease your overall volume by increasing or decreasing the lengths of your distance runs and long runs.

12-WEEK TRAINING SCHEDULE
FOR COMPETITIVE RUNNING (NEXT PHASE)
3–4 DAYS PER WEEK*

WEEK	SUN	MON	TUES	WED	THU	FRI	SAT
1	OFF	Fast Tempo-Pace Reps: 8 x 1 minute, with 2-minute jog between reps	OFF	Road Intervals: 10 x 20 seconds (sub-5K effort), with 40-second jog between reps	Distance Run or Cross Training (for equivalent time)	OFF	Long Run (include 5–10 minutes of uphill running)
2	OFF	10K-Pace Reps: 8 x 2 minutes, with 3-minute jog between reps	OFF	Hill Reps: 10 x 30 seconds, with 60-second jog/walk between reps	Distance Run or Cross Training (for equivalent time)	OFF	Long Run
3	OFF	5K-Pace Reps: 6 x 3 minutes, with 3-minute jog between reps	OFF	Hill Reps: 8 x 45 seconds, with 90-second jog/walk between reps	Distance Run or Cross Training (for equivalent time)	OFF	Long Run
4	OFF	Slow Tempo-Pace Reps: 2 x 10 minutes, with 3-minute jog between reps	OFF	Road Intervals: 15 x 30 seconds (sub-5K effort), with 60-second jog between reps	Distance Run or Cross Training (for equivalent time)	OFF	Long Run (include 5–10 minutes of uphill running)
5	OFF	10K-Pace Reps: 4 x 4 minutes, with 3-minute jog between reps	OFF	Hill Reps: 6 x 60 seconds, with 3-minute jog/walk between reps	Distance Run or Cross Training (for equivalent time)	OFF	Long Run
6	OFF	5K-Pace Reps: 4 x 4 minutes, with 3-minute jog between reps	OFF	Hill Reps: 4 x 90 seconds, with 5-minute jog/walk between reps	Distance Run or Cross Training (for equivalent time)	OFF	Long Run
7	OFF	Fast Tempo-Pace Reps: 2 x 10 minutes, with 3-minute jog between reps	OFF	Road Intervals: 20 x 30 seconds (sub-5K effort), with 60-second jog between reps	Distance Run or Cross Training (for equivalent time)	OFF	Long Run (include 5–10 minutes of uphill running)
8	OFF	10K-Pace Reps: 3 x 5 minutes, with 3-minute jog between reps	OFF	Track Workout: 12 x 200 meters (sub-5K pace), with 200m jog between reps	Distance Run or Cross Training (for equivalent time)	OFF	Long Run
9	OFF	Track Workout: 10 x 400 meters (5K pace), with 200m jog between reps	OFF	Hill Reps: 4 x 90 seconds, with 5-minute jog/walk between reps	Distance Run or Cross Training (for equivalent time)	OFF	Long Run
10	OFF	Slow Tempo-Pace Reps: 3 x 10 minutes, with 3-minute jog between reps	OFF	Road Intervals: 20 x 30 seconds (sub-5K effort), with 60-second jog between reps	Distance Run or Cross Training (for equivalent time)	OFF	Long Run (include 5–10 minutes of uphill running)
11	OFF	Track Workout: 6 x 800 meters (10K pace), with 400m jog between reps	OFF	Hill Reps: 4 x 90 seconds, with 5-minute jog/walk between reps	Distance Run or Cross Training (for equivalent time)	OFF	Long Run
12	OFF	Track Workout: 12 x 400 meters (5K pace), with 100m jog between reps	OFF	Road Intervals: 20 x 30 seconds (sub-5K effort), with 60-second jog between reps	Distance Run or Cross Training (for equivalent time)	OFF	Long Run

* For 3-day schedule, eliminate either the Wednesday or Thursday workouts.

Racing: At any point in this schedule, you can race by using either the "2-Week Training Adjustment for 5K or 10K Race" (page 117) or the "3-Week Training Adjustment for Half Marathon Race" (page 117) to prepare for your race. Then simply return to the schedule exactly where you left off.

12-WEEK TRAINING SCHEDULE
FOR COMPETITIVE RUNNING (NEXT PHASE)
5, 6, OR 7 DAYS PER WEEK*

WEEK	SUN	MON	TUES	WED	THU	FRI	SAT
1	OFF or Distance Run	Fast Tempo-Pace Reps: 8 x 1 minute, with 2-minute jog between reps	Easy Distance Run	OFF or Distance Run	Road Intervals: 10 x 20 seconds (sub-5K effort), with 40-second jog between reps	Distance Run or Cross Training (for equivalent time)	Long Run (include 5–10 minutes of uphill running)
2	OFF or Distance Run	10K-Pace Reps: 8 x 2 minutes, with 3-minute jog between reps	Easy Distance Run	OFF or Distance Run	Hill Reps: 10 x 30 seconds, with 60-second jog/walk between reps	Distance Run or Cross Training (for equivalent time)	Long Run
3	OFF or Distance Run	5K-Pace Reps: 6 x 3 minutes, with 3-minute jog between reps	Easy Distance Run	OFF or Distance Run	Hill Reps: 8 x 45 seconds, with 90-second jog/walk between reps	Distance Run or Cross Training (for equivalent time)	Long Run
4	OFF or Distance Run	Slow Tempo-Pace Reps: 2 x 10 minutes, with 3-minute jog between reps	Easy Distance Run	OFF or Distance Run	Road Intervals: 15 x 30 seconds (sub-5K effort), with 60-second jog between reps	Distance Run or Cross Training (for equivalent time)	Long Run (include 5–10 minutes of uphill running)
5	OFF or Distance Run	10K-Pace Reps: 4 x 4 minutes, with 3-minute jog between reps	Easy Distance Run	OFF or Distance Run	Hill Reps: 6 x 60 seconds, with 3-minute jog/walk between reps	Distance Run or Cross Training (for equivalent time)	Long Run
6	OFF or Distance Run	5K-Pace Reps: 4 x 4 minutes, with 3-minute jog between reps	Easy Distance Run	OFF or Distance Run	Hill Reps: 4 x 90 seconds, with 5-minute jog/walk between reps	Distance Run or Cross Training (for equivalent time)	Long Run
7	OFF or Distance Run	Fast Tempo-Pace Reps: 2 x 10 minutes, with 3-minute jog between reps	Easy Distance Run	OFF or Distance Run	Road Intervals: 8 x 60 seconds (sub-5K effort), with 60-second jog between reps	Distance Run or Cross Training (for equivalent time)	Long Run (include 5–10 minutes of uphill running)
8	OFF or Distance Run	10K-Pace Reps: 4 x 5 minutes, with 3-minute jog between reps	Easy Distance Run	OFF or Distance Run	Track Workout: 12 x 200 meters (sub-5K pace), with 200m jog between reps	Distance Run or Cross Training (for equivalent time)	Long Run
9	OFF or Distance Run	Track Workout: 10–12 x 400 meters (5K pace), with 200m jog between reps	Easy Distance Run	OFF or Distance Run	Hill Reps: 4 x 90 seconds, with 5-minute jog/walk between reps	Distance Run or Cross Training (for equivalent time)	Long Run
10	OFF or Distance Run	Slow Tempo-Pace Reps: 3 x 10 minutes, with 3-minute jog between reps	Easy Distance Run	OFF or Distance Run	Road Intervals: 10 x 60 seconds (sub-5K effort), with 60-second jog between reps	Distance Run or Cross Training (for equivalent time)	Long Run (include 5–10 minutes of uphill running)
11	OFF or Distance Run	Track Workout: 8–10 x 800 meters (10K pace), with 400m jog between reps	Easy Distance Run	OFF or Distance Run	Hill Reps: 4 x 90 seconds, with 5-minute jog/walk between reps	Distance Run or Cross Training (for equivalent time)	Long Run
12	OFF or Distance Run	Track Workout: 12–16 x 400 meters (5K pace), with 100m jog between reps	Easy Distance Run	OFF or Distance Run	Fast Tempo-Pace Reps: 4 x 5 minutes, with 2-minute jog between reps	Distance Run or Cross Training (for equivalent time)	Long Run

Racing: At any point in this schedule, you can race by using either the "2-Week Training Adjustment for 5K or 10K Race" (page 117) or the "3-Week Training Adjustment for Half Marathon Race" (page 117) to prepare for your race. Then simply return to the schedule exactly where you left off.

2-WEEK TRAINING ADJUSTMENT
FOR 5K OR 10K RACE

WEEK	SUN	MON	TUES	WED	THU	FRI	SAT
1	OFF or Distance Run (depending on your schedule)	Track Workout: 6–8 x 400 at 5K or 10K pace (whichever is your race pace), with 200m jog between reps	OFF or Easy Distance Run (depending on your schedule)	Distance Run	Easy Distance Run (50–75% normal length); include 4–8 strides (60–80 meters) at expected race pace	OFF or 20 minutes jogging	5K or 10K RACE
2	OFF or Easy Distance Run (depending on your schedule)	Distance Run	OFF or Distance Run (depending on your schedule)	Distance Run	Slow Tempo-Pace Reps: 2 x 10 minutes, with 3-minute jog between reps	OFF or Distance Run (depending on your schedule)	Long Run

3-WEEK TRAINING ADJUSTMENT
FOR HALF MARATHON RACE

WEEK	SUN	MON	TUES	WED	THU	FRI	SAT
1	OFF or Distance Run (depending on your schedule)	Fast Tempo-Pace Reps: 2 x 10 minutes, with 3-minute jog between reps	OFF or Easy Distance Run (depending on your schedule)	OFF or Distance Run (depending on your schedule)	Road Intervals: 20 x 30 seconds (sub-5K effort), with 60-second jog between reps	OFF or Distance Run (depending on your schedule)	Distance Run (regular distance-run length)
2	OFF or Distance Run (depending on your schedule)	5K-Pace Reps: 5 x 3 minutes, with 3-minute jog between reps	OFF or Easy Distance Run (depending on your schedule)	OFF or Distance Run (depending on your schedule)	Easy Distance Run (50–75% normal length); include 4–8 strides (60–80 meters) at expected race pace	OFF or 20 minutes jogging	HALF MARATHON RACE
3	OFF	Distance Run	OFF or Distance Run (depending on your schedule)	OFF or Distance Run (depending on your schedule)	Road Intervals: 10 x 20 seconds (sub-5K effort), with 40-second jog between reps	OFF or Distance Run (depending on your schedule)	Distance Run (regular distance-run length)

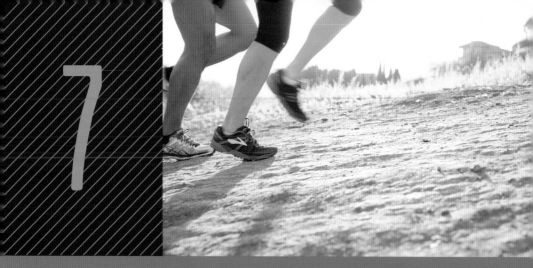

7

Shake It Up

*"You only ever grow as a human being if you're
outside your comfort zone."*

—PERCY CERUTTY

I REMEMBER MY FIRST INTERVAL WORKOUT like it was yesterday. It was summer, 1975, and I was a pint-sized, fourteen-year-old freshman on the La Cañada High School cross country team. We'd done all distance runs for the first few weeks of training, leaving from the school parking lot at 7 AM sharp, but on this particular morning, Coach Logan, an intense, type A commander in chief who scared the bejesus out of me, announced that we'd be taking a field trip. So we squeezed into a half dozen cars and drove five miles to Crescenta Valley Park, a narrow strip of grass, dirt, and cement pinched between the 210 freeway and the base of the Verdugo Mountains. The park was deserted except for our small pack, twenty-seven of us jogging, swaddled by the morning fog, our footsteps muted in dewy grass. Jeff Thompson, the team's extroverted sophomore star, seemed oddly subdued as he led us along a twisting trail and then across a bridge, spanning a cement wash, to the most remote area of the park, a several-acre pie wedge of grass and dirt that angled upward before vanishing beneath a canopy of shade trees, what Thompson called "the black forest." Thompson instructed us to stop. And then we waited. A few minutes later, Coach Logan appeared, marching toward us, stopwatch in hand. "We're running intervals," he said. I asked Randy Judd in a whisper, "What's intervals?" But Randy shushed me with a look. Logan drew a line in the dirt with his shoe, had us stand on one side of it, and said, "Go!" And off we went. The pace was fast. Really fast. I tucked behind the lead runners as we navigated a rough trail running parallel to the cement wash. And then, as we were about to run out of park, Thompson executed a sharp left turn. Like lemmings, we followed his uphill charge, heading up beneath that dark canopy. And then we were flying through the trees, first along a flat path, and then back down, a dangerously rugged plunge toward a shoestring creek, a long eyes-closed bound to clear it, and then climbing again, momentarily breaking from the black forest to ascend a final, impossibly steep dirt pitch, its upper limit marked by a solitary tree. Unbelievably, I caught Thompson at the tree, then rounded the corner ahead of him, heading back into the forest, in the lead, all the others stretched out behind me. As I exited the forest, a 100-meter strip of uneven grass between myself and Coach Logan, I let loose, my legs a whirlwind, and crossed the finish line a full 30 meters ahead of Thompson and the rest. Spent, I bent over, hands on my knees, my rib cage aching as I gobbled air. Coach Logan shook his head and scowled. "You realize," he said, "that you've got seven more reps to go." I hadn't realized that. We'd been running so fast, I'd assumed "intervals" must mean one all-out run. I thought I'd won. Instead, exhausted, my legs shaking with fatigue, I was about to endure the most painful workout of my life.

The most important thing about doing a workout is knowing *how* to do the workout correctly. And that's what this chapter is all about. We've touched on a lot of different workouts in the last two chapters (both directly and as part of the listed training for different running goals). In this chapter, we'll give the rundown on each of those workouts: its description, its purpose, and how to perform it. It's worth repeating that most of you will *not* be including all of these workouts in your personal schedules. First-time runners will have all you can handle with distance runs, stretching, basic strength work, and other lower-intensity training, even as some returning runners with ambitious race goals might want to sample higher-intensity training like speed work and plyometrics. I've put *all* the workouts into this one chapter—and have listed them alphabetically—for a simple reason: I want to make it easy for you to find the workouts that are pertinent to your training, both today and in the future (when the time comes to actually try them out). Think of this chapter as your workout encyclopedia.

TRAINING 101

Every workout has a purpose. And that purpose is *never* to annihilate you. Instead, the purpose is to challenge your body in a way that either stimulates fitness improvements or helps maintain improvements that have already occurred. Workouts that stimulate improvements should be hard enough to trigger the desired results—*and no harder*. Workouts that help maintain improvements, such as easy-paced distance runs, should always be comfortable and refreshing. A well-rounded training program will include the right mix of both types of workouts. And for the best results, it will also include a variety of each. As noted in Chapter 6, it takes a wide range of workouts to create top fitness. That's because training isn't just accumulating miles and then jotting them down in your running log. Instead, it's the process of rebuilding your running engine.

Building a better running engine

Your *running engine* is the sum total of "parts" within your body that creates and sustains your ability to run. It includes your heart, lungs, blood, blood vessels, and muscle cells. It also includes the eighty-five billion neurons in your brain and spinal cord, the nerves reaching out to every muscle in your body, and the quadrillions of messages sent every second along those nerves. It includes your hormones. And your fuel stores. And your bones, tendons, ligaments, and cartilage. It's a vast, interconnected network of dependent parts—a biological hybrid of computer and machine. And your job as a runner is to train it all.

Again, this doesn't mean that you'll be donning an exercise-scientist hat and creating a lab project out of your body. That's my job. It's simply a reminder that you should keep an open mind about including different types of running and exercises in your program. I suggest this not because I'm a stereotypical type A personality coach who enjoys seeing his athletes suffer. I suggest it because experience has shown me that a well-rounded approach is the best way to ensure uninterrupted, healthy, happy running.

The truth is that no single exercise (e.g., distance running) can target every running-engine part, any more than just doing bench presses can transform every muscle in a bodybuilder's physique. You spent the first few weeks of your running program preparing your body for the demands of training. Now, it's time to step a little bit outside your comfort zone—to challenge your fitness and to incorporate workouts that you might not have attempted (or even thought about attempting) in the past. Depending on your running goal, this might require as little as a single hard running session per week coupled with some resistance training, or as much as a multiweek schedule of distance, intervals, drills, hills, and all the rest of it.

Assembling workouts for your program

In Chapter 6, we outlined various workouts you should consider including in your program, based upon five different running goals. But we also acknowledged that many of you might have different goals—and will therefore require a unique mix of training. In creating a training schedule that includes workouts from this chapter, the following guidelines will help you to plot out the introduction of various types of training, as well as increases in volume and intensity:

FIRST 3 WEEKS: This is the pretraining period we discussed in Chapter 5, "Run First, Train Later." You'll begin with just easy walking, or easy walking paired with surges of jogging. In the second or third week, when you've become comfortable with your walking/jogging, you'll add resistance training (the Beginner's Body Strengthening routine on page 275.

WEEKS 4–6: If you're ready, you'll segue to continuous running, with a slight increase in overall volume. You'll also add strides to prepare for faster running. Runners with previous experience might move more quickly through this stage. And if weight loss is part of your long-term goal, now is the time to consider implementing your diet (although it's fine to wait a few more weeks).

WEEKS 7–9: If you're ready, you'll begin to incorporate a harder workout each week—for example, beginner's fartlek or repetitions (intervals). One run each week (usually on Saturday or Sunday) will begin to emerge as your "long run," with up to 25 percent more running scheduled for that day. Your overall volume will continue to increase.

WEEKS 10–12: If you're ready, some of you (those training for competition) will add a second hard day to your week. This run will focus on higher-intensity training, such as hill strides and hill repeats. Overall volume will continue to increase, and your long run will expand, becoming 25–50 percent longer than your regular distance runs.

BEYOND 12 WEEKS: Your volume of both endurance training (e.g., distance) and harder training (e.g., repetitions, tempo, and hill repeats) will continue to increase. Competitive runners will add workouts such as downhill running, form drills, and plyometrics to their training.

Of course, you're welcome to simply follow a sample schedule from the included training schedules—or, as mentioned in the last chapter, to stick with a distance-only program. But whether you're following a schedule from this book or creating one of your own, you'll want to become familiar with the different types of workouts available to you. And who knows, there just might come a time in the future when workouts that seem completely beyond your ability today suddenly seem doable. Don't *ever* sell yourself short—and don't ever underestimate the potential improvement you'll experience with a smart, appropriate training program.

THE WORKOUTS

While distance running provides the foundation for a strong running program, there are literally dozens of workouts that have their place in a smart, well-rounded training schedule. We'll go through the various workouts in alphabetical order—*not* in order of importance or in the order you'll introduce them into your training (this latter task being impossible since different running goals require the introduction of different workouts at different stages of training). So that you can fully understand each workout, we'll name the workout, give a brief summary of its purpose, and then explain how it's done.

Balance training

Purpose: Improves your ability to land correctly with each stride, to negotiate turns and uneven terrain, and to correct your posture and stride before injury occurs

A 2006 experiment had football players balance on each leg for five minutes, then repeat the exercise five days a week for four weeks. The result was 77 percent fewer ankle sprains during the season. While the best balance exercises involve the use of a wobble board (see page 230), you'll benefit from incorporating these three easy-to-perform exercises into your resistance training routine:

BALANCE ON ONE LEG: Stand with your knees slightly bent. Lift one foot off the floor (in front of you) and hold it. When you can't hold it any longer, put it down and repeat with the opposite leg. See page 228, for photo-instruction.

BALANCE ON ONE LEG AND BEND FORWARD: When just balancing becomes too easy, move the lifted leg behind you, straighten it, and bend down to touch your toes. Do 5–10 reps.

BALANCE ON ONE LEG WITH A MEDICINE BALL: Repeat the previous exercises while holding a medicine (or other) ball. Move the ball over your head, in front of you, and toward your toes.

Distance runs

Purpose: Distance runs strengthen your heart, increase the oxygen-carrying capacity of your blood, increase the fuel stores in your muscles, teach your body to burn more fat, and improve stride efficiency. They also strengthen your running muscles and connective tissue.

Distance runs make up the bulk of most running schedules, accounting for 80 percent or more of runners' overall running volume. They are not only the most important workouts in your program, they're also the workouts that keep most runners coming back—for the "runner's high," as an excuse to get together with friends, as a quick break from the stress of work, or simply to get outside for an hour. Four variations you'll want to slot into your program are:

JOGGING: This is running at an effort level that is just a notch above walking. New runners jog as a prerequisite for running. And experienced runners jog as part of their warm-up or cool-down.

EASY DISTANCE RUN: This is a low-intensity run that's perfect for the early stages of a running program and for recovery days later in your program.

REGULAR DISTANCE RUN: Your bread-and-butter distance run. The pace should be conversational.

LONG RUN: The long run can account for up to 35–45 percent of the week's volume for runners training 3–4 days per week, and 20–25 percent for those training 5–7 days. After approximately 90 minutes of running, you start building new capillaries (small blood vessels around your muscle cells) and burning extra fat. Because long runs are the weekly focal point for many running groups, this workout is central to creating the sense of fraternity that exists among the men and women in the sport.

Downhill running

Purpose: Downhill running increases the workload on your front thighs (quadriceps), triggering greater strength adaptations in those muscles.

This isn't a workout for inexperienced runners. But it's a *great* workout for runners interested in increasing their speed or running a race that includes downhill segments (e.g., the Boston Marathon). It's also a terrific cure for chronic quadriceps pain, which is why you'll find it explained in the Injury-Prevention Exercises on page 261. For experienced runners, downhill running is a nice change of pace from weekly hill reps, speed work, or drills.

Fartlek

Purpose: Fartlek is Swedish for "speed play." The mix of intensities targets your cardiovascular system, your full range of muscle cells, and your nervous system. It's the best all-around tune-up for your running engine.

In fartlek, you alternate easy running with harder surges that last between 20 seconds and 3 minutes. The decision of when to surge and recover (and for how long to do each) is made on the fly. This is a great early workout for runners segueing from the first three weeks of running to more advanced training. And, in case you're wondering, no, you're not the first person in the history of running to snort and giggle at the word fartlek.

FARTLEK: After warming up, begin with a series of moderate-effort surges, each lasting 10–20 seconds followed by 30–60 seconds of jogging. Next, alternate surges of various duration and intensity with recovery periods of walking, jogging, or easy running—the idea is to recover almost completely after each surge. Faster surges (e.g., 1-mile race pace) should be limited to between 20 and 30 seconds. Slower surges (e.g., 5K race pace) can last for 1–3 minutes. Recovery periods can last from 30 seconds to 5 minutes. You can do this workout on roads, trails, or grass—or all three. The actual fartlek session should last 10–30 minutes.

BEGINNER'S FARTLEK: This workout is conducted just like regular fartlek, except that you limit your faster surges to between 10 and 15 seconds and your slower surges to between 20 and 60 seconds.

Form drills

Purpose: Drills lengthen your stride, increase your stride rate (the number of strides you take per minute), improve nervous system efficiency, and increase your overall speed.

When you think of your stride, you probably think of one single motion. But your stride is actually a chain of actions strung together—foot contact, push-off, backswing, forward swing, knee lift, and more. Drills isolate each link in that chain and then train it, improving nervous system control of each action and strengthening the muscles and connective tissue involved. Experienced runners make drills a regular part of their training (see my book *Build Your Running Body* for a complete routine). For most novice runners, however, drills aren't advised; you're still developing your stride through basic training (see the entry "Stride work" in this chapter). That said, if your running goal is to compete, you'll want to work three drills into your warm-up (before harder workouts) once or twice a week, beginning in week nine or ten. Follow each drill by jogging back to your start line, then running a moderate-intensity stride for the same distance. Walk back to the start as recovery before your next drill.

SKIPPING: Yes, just like you did back in the schoolyard. Take off on one foot, land on the same foot, then switch to the other. Repeat. Skip 20–60 meters.

FLAT-FOOTED MARCHING: Stand tall and start marching forward. Lift your knee to at least hip height while keeping your opposite foot flat on the ground. Then bring your lifted foot down, using a flat-footed plant. Repeat with the opposite knee. March for 20–60 meters.

BUTT KICKS: Stay on the balls of your feet, running tall, and alternately kick your heels back toward your glutes (butt). Keep your thighs perpendicular to the ground. Perform for 20–60 meters.

Hill repeats

Purpose: Hill repeats strengthen all your muscle cells—especially those that generate speed and power. They also increase your ability to produce aerobic energy at faster paces (by a lot!).

Hill repetitions are what they sound like: running up a hill multiple times. You'll want to find a hill that's challenging, but not so steep that you can't maintain a good stride—anywhere from a 3–6 percent grade is fine. Make sure to include a few hills in your distance runs before progressing to hill repeats. Hill repeats aren't for your first few weeks of training. Instead, wait until you're ready to add a second hard workout to your week, or at least until you've mastered repetitions and tempo training. Hill repeats are the best running workout for building your power—your ability to drive up a hill or to maintain a fast pace on level ground for a sustained period of time.

HILL STRIDES: Hill strides should last 10–20 seconds (no longer), and should be run at about 90 percent effort (not an all-out sprint). For recovery, walk back down the hill, allowing 1–3 minutes between reps. Start with 4–5 reps and build up to 10.

HILL REPEATS: Run up a hill for 30–90 seconds at an effort that's "hard," but not so hard that you struggle to complete the workout. For recovery, jog down the hill and then walk at the bottom until your recovery period is over. Each week, add time to both your repetitions and your recovery. A typical week-to-week workout progression would be:

→ 6–10 x 30 seconds, with 60-second recovery

→ 4–8 x 60 seconds, with 3-minute recovery

→ 3–6 x 90 seconds, with 5-minute recovery

Plyometrics

Purpose: Plyometric exercises improve the explosive power of your muscles, your elastic recoil, and your running economy.

Plyometrics are exercises that require short, maximum efforts from your muscles—*and* they're a type of training that most of you will skip for now (as with form drills, see my book *Build Your Running Body* for a full complement of plyometric exercises). For those runners hell-bent on kicking a— and taking names, however, here are two basic plyometric drills that can be worked into your resistance training routine:

DOUBLE-LEG HOPS: Stand with your feet hip-width apart. Then squat as you pull your arms down and behind you. When your quads are parallel to the ground, explode upward, leaping as high as you can go. Let your knees bend as you land, absorbing the impact force, and then (this is the important part) spring upward again. Continue for 3–5 total jumps.

QUICK HOPS: Start with both feet hip-width apart, a slight bend at your knees. Jump forward with both feet, but stay low to the ground. You don't want height. You want a quick succession of short jumps, using both feet to jump and land. Hop for 15–25 meters.

You should *never* attempt plyometrics until you have at least three weeks of resistance training under your belt.

Repetitions (also called "Intervals")

Purpose: Repetitions increase your heart's pumping capacity, strengthen your running muscles, increase your ability to produce aerobic energy, improve running economy (at the paces run during the workout), and stimulate multiple other positive adaptations.

This workout is called "repetitions" by some, "intervals" by others. In it, you alternate fixed periods of harder running with periods of jogging, walking, or standing. Technically, the periods of harder running are the *repetitions,* and the recovery periods are the *intervals.* The repetitions are run at various effort levels known to stimulate positive changes in your fitness. The rest intervals allow you to recover, increasing the amount of work you can do at the beneficial effort level. Since different paces stimulate different benefits, a well-rounded program includes repetitions at multiple paces. Most runners schedule repetition workouts during their first months of training. And almost all runners who plan to race prepare with repetitions at their expected race pace. Repetitions are *always* preceded by a full warm-up (at least 15 minutes of jogging and some strides). Repetition workouts included in this book's training schedules include:

30-SECOND REPETITIONS: You run hard (a little faster than 5K race pace) for 30 seconds, then immediately slow to a walk or jog for 60 seconds. Then repeat 10–20 times. This workout dates to the late 1930s, when Woldemar Gerschler and Hans Reindell conducted a study with three thousand participants. After three weeks of training, the participants averaged a 20 percent increase in heart volume. That translates to more blood pumped with each heartbeat, which means more oxygen delivered to your muscles and, subsequently, more aerobic energy.

ROAD & TRAIL REPETITIONS: These repetitions are run at a pace that approximates either a 5K or 10K race effort. Repetitions last between 1 and 5 minutes, with a recovery jog of 2–3 minutes between repetitions. If you don't know your 5K or 10K pace, simply run at an effort level that allows you to complete the workout feeling fatigued but not destroyed.

TRACK REPETITIONS: These repetitions are run on a 400-meter track. The length of the repetition is set by distance (not time, as with road and trail reps), a goal time is targeted for each rep, and the recovery interval can be given as either a distance (e.g., 200 meters of jogging) or a time (e.g., 1 minute of jogging). An example of this type of workout would be: 12 x 400 meters at goal 5K pace, with 200 meters of jogging between repetitions.

Resistance training

Purpose: Resistance training increases explosive power in your legs, improves all-around muscle balance (reducing the chance of injury), and improves running economy.

Resistance training will build your muscular strength through exercises that force you to work against an opposing force (this can be your own body weight, free weights, resistance bands, or machines). It's also been shown to improve running itself. A 2015 study published in the *International Journal of Sports Physiology and Performance* found that six weeks of resistance training "significantly improves 5-km time." And a 2013 study concluded that resistance training improves running economy in masters marathoners by 6 percent, again after only six weeks. This book offers a Beginner's Body Strengthening routine on page 275. You might also incorporate some of the exercises highlighted following Chapter 12's injury-prevention instruction. Most runners will benefit from one or two sessions of resistance training per week, beginning the second or third week of your running program.

Speed work

Purpose: Speed work teaches your body to run at very fast paces. Your nervous system learns how to activate your full range of muscle cells—in the process strengthening them—and your body becomes better able to utilize anaerobic energy. It also improves running economy.

While some runners consider all repetition workouts to be "speed work," we'll limit our definition of these workouts to hill sprints and track repetitions at mile race pace or faster. Like drills and plyometrics, these aren't workouts that most novice runners will include in their programs. Competitive runners with at least ten weeks of training under their belts can consider substituting these workouts for their second hard training session of each week. Speed work (especially hill sprints) improves running efficiency for all races from the mile to the marathon.

HILL SPRINTS: Find a fairly steep hill (approximately a 6–8 percent grade), then sprint up it at 90–95 percent maximum effort for 6–12 seconds (no longer). Walk down the hill, resting for at least 1 minute and as many as 3. Start with 4 reps and, over subsequent workouts, build up to 8.

TRACK 150S & 200S: Run fast repetitions on a local track. For 150-meter repetitions, run 4–6 reps at a pace you could maintain for 800 meters, then walk/jog for 250 meters. For 200-meter repetitions, run 6–12 reps at 1-mile race pace, then walk/jog for 200 meters.

Stretching

Purpose: Active isolated stretching improves your muscles' range of motion, dynamic stretching prepares your muscles for running, and static stretching relieves stiffness post-run.

All stretching is not the same. When a 2012 Croatian research project, which reviewed more than one hundred studies on stretching, concluded that pre-run static stretching reduces strength by 5 percent and explosive power by 3 percent (for that workout—not permanently), many runners were ready to ditch stretching for good. Don't. Just use the correct type of stretching during different phases of your workout.

DYNAMIC STRETCHING: Controlled leg swings increase your muscles' range of motion and activate your muscles. Do *before* hard workouts as part of your warm-up (after jogging). See "Leg swings" (page 238).

STATIC STRETCHING: Hold a position that stretches the muscle. Static stretching performed immediately post-run relieves stiffness, leaving you loose for the next day's run. See "Hamstring static stretch" (page 254), "Calf static stretch" (page 255) and "Hip flexors stretch" (page 244).

ACTIVE ISOLATED STRETCHING (AIS): You use an opposing muscle to move a muscle into a stretched position (e.g., you flex your quadriceps muscle to lift your leg, stretching your hamstring), then slightly increase the stretch by applying a 1- or 2-second gentle pull with a rope. AIS can be incorporated into your resistance training routine. See "AIS calves" (page 226) and "AIS hamstrings" (page 242).

Strides

Purpose: Strides work all your muscle cells, help hone and maintain nervous system control of your muscle fibers, and prepare your body for faster, longer efforts.

Strides are a safe and fun way for new runners to work their faster muscle cells (intermediate fast-twitch and fast-twitch), for experienced runners to reinforce muscle and nervous system adaptations from training, and for all runners to prepare for harder efforts (higher-intensity training sessions, such as repetitions, and races). A stride is a brief acceleration to "fast" running. Fast doesn't mean an all-out sprint. Instead, you'll build up to an 80–95 percent maximum speed for a duration of 5–20 seconds (anywhere from 30 to 100+ meters), with speed and duration determined both by your fitness and whether the strides are a workout or a part of your warm-up.

WORKOUT STRIDES: You'll run anywhere from 4–10 strides either during your workout (after at least 10 minutes of easy jogging or running for a warm-up) or post-workout. Between each stride, you'll jog slowly for an equivalent distance. New runners will accelerate to 80–85 percent of their maximum speed, while experienced runners might shoot for as much as 95 percent of their maximum speed.

WARM-UP STRIDES: When warming up for either a harder workout (e.g., repetitions or hill repeats) or a race, strides help to prepare your body for the effort. You'll do 4–8 strides, building up to a pace equivalent to what you expect to run during the workout/race. This helps to prepare your body for a longer effort at that pace.

Stride work

We touched on this back in Chapter 4 (under "Bad form"). As a runner, you'll hear a lot about adjusting your stride. And there's a huge market for selling you form fixes. Shoes offer "motion control." Books and classes promise to teach you a better stride. And running gurus suggest that you can harness gravity (i.e., you can fall forward rather than having to bother pushing off with your feet), an assumption to which physicist and *Runner's World* columnist Alex Hutchinson replies, "But the claim that gravity—a force directed straight downward—gives you free energy to help travel in a forward direction is simply wrong." Look, when you start running, you have a beginner's stride. This is not the stride you'll have in a few months. So be patient. Let all your distance runs, repetitions, tempo work, and resistance training do their magic. If you include drills and plyometrics in your training, allow those exercises to naturally strengthen all aspects of your stride. Better fitness, stronger muscles, and a more efficient nervous system will do wonders for your running form. Attempting to willfully alter your stride—to assume conscious control of up to seventeen quadrillion nerve impulses per second—is a fool's errand. If, after a few months, you still have some obvious form malfunction (e.g., landing with your foot in front of your body, known as "overstriding"), then find a local coach with solid credentials (i.e., he or she has coached a club, school, or successful individual runners) to help work on modest adjustments.

Tempo runs

Purpose: A tempo run improves oxygen delivery to muscle cells, aerobic energy production, and your ability to maintain effort (pace) during slightly anaerobic conditions (such as those that occur during distance races from 5K to the marathon).

Tempo is one of the most popular and misunderstood workouts in running. This is what tempo is *not*: a time trial (an all-out effort for the scheduled distance). Instead, tempo is run at an effort that über-coach Jack Daniels, author of *Daniels' Running Formula*, calls "comfortably hard." For Daniels, tempo is equivalent to the maximum pace a runner can maintain for one hour. I prefer slightly less challenging paces for tempo, somewhere between half marathon and marathon pace (less chance of overtraining that way). Running harder than correct tempo effort won't get you fit faster. Instead, it will simply lengthen the time (days) it takes you to recover. Tempo is a valuable workout for all runners, although you'll want to wait eight to ten weeks before working it into your program. Tempo should always be preceded by a full warm-up.

TEMPO REPETITIONS: I prefer tempo repetitions to continuous tempo running. That's because, no matter our intention, we runners still tend to run tempo too hard. Breaking the workout into repetitions allows us to settle down during the recovery interval, re-gauge our effort, and finish the workout at the correct effort level. Repetitions should last 5–10 minutes, with a 3-minute jog recovery between reps, for a total volume of 10–20 minutes (fast tempo pace) or 15–30 minutes (slow tempo pace).

FAST TEMPO: 10–20 minutes of continuous running at half marathon effort.

SLOW TEMPO: 15–30 minutes of continuous running at marathon effort.

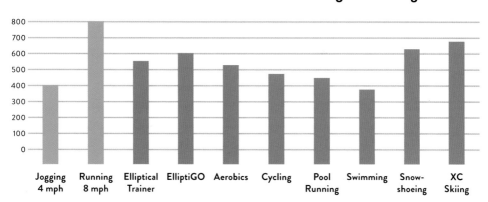

Calories Burned: 1 Hour of Cross Training vs. Running

CROSS TRAINING

Cross training refers to non-running exercises. While cross training can and *should* be a big part of your program, it's important to understand that no non-running exercise can ever deliver the same fitness benefits for your running as, well, *running*. Back in Chapter 2, we discussed "specificity of training"—the fact that you improve most at specific types of exercise by doing that exercise. Cross training fails the specificity of exercise test. But don't despair. Some cross training exercises don't fail by that much (i.e., they target many of the same muscles and movements as running, just not all of them), and they improve your overall fitness in other ways. Here are some good reasons to include cross training in your program, beginning as early as your first few weeks of running:

→ You strengthen your heart without sustaining additional foot-strike impact. While some impact is good for strengthening muscles and connective tissue, too much can lead to injury.

→ For exercises that closely mimic running (e.g., the elliptical machine and snowshoeing), you add volume to your schedule without adding foot-strike impact.

→ It's a good substitute for running when you're injured.

→ If you're not ready to run, it's a *great* way to experience the thrill of a run. You can hop on an ElliptiGO bike or an elliptical machine and get a taste of the running experience.

As the chart, "Calories Burned: 1 Hour of Cross Training vs. Running," illustrates, most cross training activities require about the same physical intensity (measured in calories burned) as jogging or running. Some of the best cross training activities for runners are listed below.

Treadmill

This is as close as you can get to running outdoors without being, you know, outdoors—a godsend when severe weather makes normal running impossible (or at least impractical). Be aware that you'll use a slightly different stride, overheat a little quicker (due to the lack of any breeze), and run a little slower than on the roads or trails (up to two minutes per mile for some runners).

Elliptical trainer

This machine allows you to mimic the act of walking or running, minus the impact. Some models include moveable handles so that you can work your upper body.

ElliptiGO bicycle

This is an elliptical machine that's also a bike. The handles are stationary, but other than that, this is the closest you'll come to mimicking an outdoor run without actually running.

Pool running

A terrific cross training exercise for runners. Use an AquaJogger (or other) buoyancy belt, make sure your feet don't touch the bottom of the pool, and then move your legs just like you would on the road. You can simulate distance, tempo, or even repetitions.

Snowshoeing

A great option for those who live in the snow. Because snowshoeing is physically demanding—and really tough the first couple times out—do your initial sessions on flat terrain. And don't be shy about taking walk breaks.

Cross-country skiing

Maybe the best workout there is for increasing your ability to create aerobic energy. Both classic skiing and skate skiing will give you a good workout.

Aerobics class

A catch-all phrase for dancing, spinning, step aerobics, martial arts, stair-climbing, and other classes that remain favorites at many gyms. A vibrant social atmosphere for runners interested in all-around fitness.

Cycling

You can go farther and faster cycling (stationary bikes excluded) than you can by running, but you use significantly different muscle cells than you do running. Cycling's fun, but it's less helpful for running than other cross training choices.

Swimming

Freestyle and butterfly are the best strokes for cross training, but no stroke is directly applicable to running. If you start to sink, ask a coach or experienced swimmer how to "press the T" in order to remain buoyant.

BECOMING A RUNNER: *Luis Palacios*

Luis Palacios emigrated from Mexico to the United States in 2006, at age twenty-seven. He'd never envisioned a move north of the border. But on a visit to his dentist, in Tijuana, Mexico, he'd noticed a young woman, Jennifer, pacing the clinic halls, entering and exiting the building. He asked her, in Spanish, if she was lost. And Jennifer answered in broken Spanish that she couldn't find the lot where she'd parked her car. Luis helped her, one thing led to another, and they were soon married. They moved to Jennifer's home in Dana Point, California. "And I didn't have anything to do," says Luis. "I didn't have friends. No family. My wife was working." Luis couldn't speak English yet—though he was taking ESL classes—and couldn't put the medical degree he'd earned from the University of Sinaloa, in Sinaloa, Mexico, to use, so he felt isolated and alone: "It was horrible. I was miserable." And so, with no previous athletic training of any kind, he decided to try jogging. After all, it didn't require friends or English. First, he jogged a couple times a week. Then a little more. And by the end of his first year, he was training five days a week and getting more sophisticated. "I started running with mile markers," he says. "I had a bike and an odometer, and I'd put tape on walls or fences. I had a little loop, and with my watch I could keep track of the pace." Eventually, Luis would discover that all

When you create a smart, sustainable, and effective running program, you aren't just making a list of workouts and then entering them into a training log. I mean, sure, that's part of the process. But that's not what you're doing. *Not really.* What you're really doing is beginning construction on an entirely new you.

You're laying out the blueprint to build a new body.

And to forge a new mentality.

We've outlined a lot of workouts in this chapter. There's a reason for that. Just as a surgeon wouldn't operate without the proper instruments,

his mile markers were off, but by then he'd switched to training by heart rate. In 2008, Luis ran his first 5K. "I ended up winning the race!" he says. His training took another leap forward when he met Juan Luis Barrios, one of Mexico's top distance runners, at a race in Carlsbad, California, and struck up a friendship. Barrios recommended higher mileage and other advanced training. Shortly thereafter, Luis dropped his 5K personal best all the way to 15:55. At the same time, it was getting harder to find the necessary hours to train. Since becoming a full-time employee at the trauma unit for Mission Hospital (Mission Viejo), in 2009, and with two children, Sariah and Andreas, Luis had been rising at 4:30 AM to get in his runs. When he began to prepare for his medical board exams, in order to practice as a doctor in the United States, something had to give. So he once again shifted his running goals, this time away from competitive running and back toward an emphasis on an active, fit lifestyle. "Until I finish my boards," says Luis, "running is just about staying healthy." He adds, "Of course, my goal is to keep running until I'm old, very old."

or a mechanic without the right tools, you'll need the correct workouts to build a body that can achieve your running goals.

At a running seminar, I was once asked, "What are the best workouts for becoming a better runner?" I answered, without hesitation, "The ones whose purpose you understand and that you know how to do correctly."

A runner with a pocketful of workouts that he or she can execute correctly, and that will trigger the desired fitness improvements, is well-armed, indeed.

Choose your workouts wisely. Be patient. Persevere. And you'll soon be a fit runner.

CHAPTER TAKEAWAY

Before you begin a workout, you should know two things: why you're doing the workout, and how to do the workout. Every workout has a purpose, and runners need to know what those purposes are before they begin entering workouts into their schedules. If you think of your body as a running engine, the different parts would be your heart, lungs, blood, muscles, bones, tendons, nerves, etc. Good training involves scheduling workouts that target, train, and improve all those parts. While some runners can get by on a diet of distance, repetitions, and resistance training, others will want to sample the smorgasbord of available workouts in order to build the best running body possible.

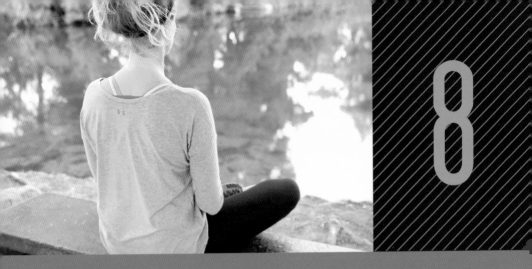

The No-Mistake Zone

"Reality is that which, when you stop believing in it, doesn't go away."

—PHILIP K. DICK

NO ONE SETS OUT TO TRAIN INCORRECTLY. We set out to get fit. To lose weight. To de-stress. To steer for some beacon of health or wellness that we envision in our future. Sure, some runners chase get-fit-quick schemes (and we'll identify a few variations of these in this chapter). But certainly that's not you. After all, you're reading this book. You've read the last three chapters and embraced the mantra of patience, perseverance, and proper training. So what could possibly go wrong?

In a word: *everything.*

Because you're human. And as a human, you've inherited a legacy of mistake-prone behavior. We misplace our keys, forget birthdays, oversleep, eat poorly, drink too much, get sunburned, get lost, bounce checks, date ~~narcissists delinquents lunatics~~ people with whom we're incompatible, send text messages to the wrong recipient, misplace passwords (or never write them down), miss garbage day, honk in traffic jams, vote for criminals, and, seriously, do I need to go on? Personally, back in high school, I wore an Angel's Flight form-fitting disco suit to the Spring Formal—and thought I looked spectacular.

So, if you're like pretty much every other runner on the planet, you can expect to make a few running mistakes, too. In fact, if you're like me, you can expect to make a *lot* of them. In the four decades since I went for my first run, I can honestly say that I've made *every single mistake* in this chapter. While it's easy to see some mistakes coming from a mile away, others are more insidious—they sneak up on you, cloaked in common sense, suggested by running partners, peddled under the guise of "expertise" by running publications, and often whispering the seemingly innocuous come-on: *Just this once can't hurt. . . .*

This chapter will introduce you to fifteen of these potential mistakes. We'll begin with a few that are simply counterproductive, then count down to those that are out-and-out lethal. Along the way, we'll explore strategies for avoiding each.

THE NO-MISTAKE ZONE

I tell my athletes that running is a *no-mistake zone.* Any mistake you make, you pay for. That payment will be extracted via strained muscles, inflamed tendons, stress fractures, and a fried nervous system, among other potential manifestations of physical and mental breakdown. There are no free passes, and it only takes letting your guard down once—one overexuberant distance run, one overly ambitious repetitions workout, one skipped recovery day, one set of strides in the wrong shoes (or in no shoes), one thing we thought we could get away with (but can't)—to derail months of careful, correct, incremental training.

LEARNING TO LAUGH AT OURSELVES

"If you never have a 'bad' day, you're probably doing something wrong; if you never have a 'good' day, you're definitely doing something wrong."

—Mark Remy, *Runner's World* columnist and author of *The Runner's Rule Book*, among others

The first step in avoiding mistakes is to identify them. The next step is obvious, but it bears putting into words: Once the mistakes are identified, make a commitment to keeping them out of your program.

Mistake 15: Breathing patterns

You'd think we'd trust our bodies when it comes to breathing. After all, evolution outfitted us with both conscious and subconscious control of our lungs to ensure a steady supply of oxygen—whether tracking prey during ancient persistence hunts or napping like a baby during a Sunday afternoon football game. But some runners can't leave breathing alone. And, sooner or later, they're going to suggest that you don't, either. You'll hear that you need to adopt a specific breathing pattern, synchronizing inhalation and exhalation with your strides. For instance, in a 2:2 pattern, you inhale for two strides, then exhale for two. A 3:2 pattern is also popular. This is supposed to maximize oxygen intake and stabilize your core. A study, "Running and breathing in mammals," favors a 2:1 pattern, but also notes that humans adopt patterns of 4:1, 3:1, 1:1, and 5:2. Other experts suggest 3:3 and 2:3 as options. Only one thing is certain: None of these breathing patterns will actually increase the amount of oxygen that reaches your bloodstream, but experimenting with them when you should be focusing on running just might drive you bonkers.

Avoid this mistake: Just breathe. Left alone, you'll adopt a pattern that works just fine—or maybe you won't, which is OK, too, since studies show that humans don't require regimented breathing patterns to exercise. Also, understand that you're getting enough oxygen already. The trick isn't getting more oxygen into your lungs; it's getting it into your bloodstream, which requires workouts (e.g., repetitions) that expand your battalion of oxygen-carrying red blood cells and your inventory of muscle-based aerobic power plants. Oh, and don't use nasal strips, either; you should be breathing through your mouth, not your nose.

Mistake 14: Shiny objects

We runners love our high-tech gadgetry. We buy GPS watches to measure distance and pace. Heart-rate monitors to gauge our effort. And fitness trackers to count every step we take, calorie we eat, and minute we sleep. So naturally you're disappointed when your GPS tells you you're five seconds per mile slower on this week's long run than last week's. Or when a workout in your heart rate monitor's "recovery zone" leaves you gasping for air. Or when your weight goes up even as your fitness tracker assures you that you're eating 500 fewer calories per day. *What's going on?* What's going on is that you've placed your faith in gadgets that lack the capacity to measure your training accurately. For example . . .

GPS WATCH: You ran 3.56 miles in 31 minutes and 15 seconds—27 seconds slower than last week. You're bummed. Then again, you did run with a brace on your ankle, a result of that slight sprain during one-on-one basketball last weekend. And you ran in the rain. In your basketball high-tops (left your trainers at the gym again). With a cold. At night. Without your glasses (left them on the kitchen table). Against the wind. After skipping dinner, the result of a fight with your spouse over whether you care more about running than her (or him).

HEART-RATE MONITOR: Uh-oh, you just exceeded your maximum heart rate. *Are you dead?* No, you're not. Formulas for determining max heart rate are notoriously inaccurate. So are heart-rate zones, given that everyone's zone is slightly different. And given that proper training changes the range for each zone. Also, heart rate is affected by outdoor temperature, work stress, lack of sleep, dehydration, caffeine, etc.

FITNESS TRACKER: You walk 10,000 steps every day. Eat 2,400 calories per day, as recommended. And sleep 7.5 hours per night. *So why did you gain two pounds, lose to an eight-year-old boy in last Saturday's 5K, and need a triple shot of espresso to stay awake on Monday at work?* Maybe because a 2014 study found average error ratings of more than 10 percent for fitness trackers. And because you're a real person and not an average of all people your age, weight, and gender (i.e., the recommended numbers don't apply to you personally—or, really, to anyone).

Avoid this mistake: There's a place for gadgets in your running program. You can measure out new runs. Time repetitions. Maintain a general overview of all the factors gadgets claim to measure. But an overreliance on these gadgets—and the data they provide, absent any context—won't make you a better-informed runner. It will divorce you from the real-world variables that play into every workout (everything from hangover fatigue from yesterday's workout to today's weather to the diet soda you had with lunch). Your fitness decision-making should result from a combination of rational scheduling, listening to your body, and, finally, objective feedback. It should not be dictated by measurements offered up by shiny objects.

Mistake 13: Resistance to change

Some days, our bodies just aren't up to the workout we've scheduled. On those days, smart runners change their workouts. Soon-to-be-exhausted (or possibly injured) runners don't. Just as your GPS and heart-rate monitor aren't accurate ways to measure the value of a workout, a pre-determined distance, pace, or other effort shouldn't override real-world feedback while you're exercising. A good workout isn't defined by what you write in your running log; it's determined by its effect on your body—and on your ability to recover and rebuild afterward.

Avoid this mistake: If your body isn't up to a workout, change the workout. Flexibility when executing your schedule is essential for healthy training. "A huge mistake athletes make is their inability to adjust workouts on the fly," says Christian Cushing-murray, a clubmate of mine, as well as a former 3:55 miler and current high school distance coach. "The best thing [Santa Monica Track Club coach] Joe Douglas ever did for me was to *not* tell me what the workout was going to be. If we were doing quarter repeats, he'd never tell us how many. It allowed him to adjust—if he saw you were tired that day—without having to worry that you'd feel like you were failing."

Mistake 12: Post-run refueling

So you finish a workout. Stretch. Do some post-run exercises. Take a shower. Get dressed. Then start preparing a nice meal—breakfast, lunch, or dinner, depending on when you ran. Congratulations. You just blew your recovery. You have a fifteen- to thirty-minute window post-run to ingest a carbohydrate and protein supplement if you want to speed recovery and restock your muscle cells' internal fuel source for the next day's workout.

Avoid this mistake: Treat yourself to a carbohydrate and protein snack within the first 15 minutes post-workout. Use a 3:1 or 4:1 ratio of carbs to protein. Shoot for 200–500 calories total, depending on the length of your workout.

Post-Workout Recovery Options

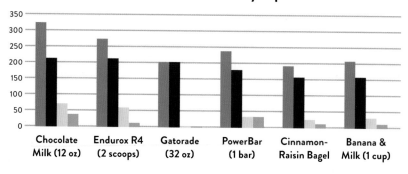

Mistake 11: No pain, no gain

"No pain, no gain" may be the most famous training slogan in the history of sports. But it's also the most destructive. Besides the fact that it's simply incorrect, *no pain, no gain* implies a tempting quid pro quo: If you *do* exercise to the point of pain, you *will* gain. In a culture obsessed with instant gratification, that's a deal most wannabe athletes are ready to make. Of course, the reality is that, more times than not, all *no pain, no gain* gets you is this: pain.

Avoid this mistake: Remember that you create changes in your body by doing the correct amount of exercise at the correct effort level. More doesn't get you fitter. It just lengthens the amount of time you'll need to recover—and it risks injury toward no end. You wouldn't pay twenty dollars for a three-dollar cup of coffee, and you shouldn't exercise to the point of pain when an exhilarating and manageable workout will net you the same result.

Mistake 10: Running fundamentalism

Running fundamentalists (RFs) are runners (often masters runners) who become set in their ways. RFs have zero interest in trying new training programs or workouts. Instead, they settle on a few workouts they like—in the case of experienced runners, usually routines that worked in the past—even when those workouts lose their effectiveness. As far as RFs are concerned: *If it worked once, it will work again.* But there's a reason it worked once. When you first begin to train, any running (as long as it's not so hard that it leads to injury) will make you a better runner. That's what your body does. It adapts! And that's a hard first impression to shake. So RFs repeat a cycle of training that no longer leads to improvement and instead triggers stagnant performances, overuse injuries, and the inevitable time off to heal.

Avoid this mistake: As your body changes, your training must change. And, for the record, your body changes constantly. It changes with age, diet, lifestyle, injury, weight, stress, illness, etc. More to the point, it changes with training. Every time you complete a workout, it changes a little. When you complete a series of workouts—when you stick to a running program over the course of weeks, months, or even years—you rebuild your body completely. When your body isn't static, your training can't be static, either.

Mistake 9: Cafeteria training

Scott Douglas, of *Runner's World*, coined this term for runners who treat training like a smorgasbord. "They are the ones who choose the elements they find most appealing from a million sources and then cram them all into a week," says Douglas. "Brad Hudson says to do hill sprints, Magill says to do drills, Jack Daniels says twenty-minute tempos, Solinsky does rhythm runs, plus I gotta do my long run, and I hear it's good to finish those with one-minute pickups!" Cafeteria trainers are searching for the training equivalent of a multivitamin. And with twenty-three hours every day between runs, they have lots of time for their search—time for the tireless over-thinker in their cerebral cortex to scavenge interesting-sounding workouts from websites, magazines, books, and other runners, and which an impulsive prefrontal cortex then schedules one after another, much like a child ripping open presents on Christmas morning. The result is almost always sore muscles, fatigue, disappointing results, injury, and a trip back to the couch.

Avoid this mistake: Don't scavenge workouts from multiple training programs. While different coaches prefer different workouts to create running fitness, most of those workouts target the same systems. Doing multiple versions of the same workout won't increase your odds of developing all-around fitness; instead, it will overwhelm the targeted systems. Until you're confident in your ability to assemble workouts that will carry you to your fitness goal, stick with one program from one source at a time.

Mistake 8: Goal fitness

Runners who plan on racing make this mistake more than any other: They base their workouts on the fitness they'd like to have rather than the fitness they actually possess. If their goal race is a marathon, they train distance at their predicted marathon pace. If it's a 5K, they do repetitions based upon their hoped-for 5K time. They do this even when they're nowhere near goal fitness. They believe that running at goal pace somehow teaches their body to complete an entire race at that pace, as if the pace seeps directly into their muscles and bones and nerves. But it doesn't. Calling a training pace "race pace" doesn't guarantee that you'll ever run that pace in an actual race. If it did, every American high school boy who ran 200-meter repetitions in sub-30 seconds (thousands every year) and called it "mile pace" would become a sub-4-minute miler (only nine have ever done that). Or every runner who trained at 5K race pace but called it marathon pace would be able to last 26.2 miles instead of only 3.1.

Avoid this mistake: Your body doesn't create major fitness improvements in response to goal pace training. It adapts in response to the demand that exercise places on muscles, energy systems, your nervous system, and more. It's true that certain *current* race paces (as in, the pace you're capable of if you raced today) are associated with specific improvements—for example, repetitions and tempo runs based upon current race paces trigger big gains in your ability to produce aerobic energy. But that's not the same as training at a pace that your body, in its current shape, cannot maintain. That won't lead to better racing. It will lead to shortened workouts and excessive fatigue. Build a better running body, and faster race paces will come. (Note: Once you've reached goal fitness, it's a different story; at that point, workouts at goal race pace will improve your running efficiency at that pace.)

Mistake 7: Stride adjustments

We've covered this twice already (see Chapter 4, page 50, and Chapter 7, page 132). So we won't repeat all the reasons that consciously attempting to change your stride is a bad idea. Instead, we'll just repeat one: The stride you have when you begin training is not the stride you'll have in a few months. Making changes early in your training is not only unnecessary, it's counterproductive.

Avoid this mistake: Wait a few months, then take your new stride for a test drive. Spend those months doing distance runs, repetitions, and resistance training, as well as drills and plyometrics if your stride is a major concern. If you're still dissatisfied with your stride, seek out a knowledgeable coach for hands-on instruction. In the meantime, understand a "great stride" isn't a visual description; it's a functional one.

Mistake 6: High-intensity interval training (HIIT)

High-intensity interval training (HIIT) isn't a mistake in itself. In fact, HIIT is an essential element of a competitive running program. The operative word is "element." HIIT actually encompasses a wide range of workouts, including both traditional repetitions (e.g., 400-meter reps on the track) and a new breed of super-short, super-high-intensity repetitions followed by limited recovery intervals (e.g., "Tabata intervals," which call for 20 seconds of maximum-effort exercise followed by a 10-second rest interval, repeated 7–8 times). This latter type of training has been embraced by many popular fitness programs, which claim Tabata-type HIIT produces all the benefits of traditional endurance training in a fraction of the time. Which is half-true. It *does* improve your ability to produce aerobic energy, but the improvement is both short-lived and inferior to that created through traditional training. You'll max out on benefits in six to eight weeks of training, after which the nervous system fatigue and stress on your muscles can lead to diminished performance, reduced motivation, and the possibility of injury.

Avoid this mistake: Limit HIIT (e.g., hill sprints and speed work) to sessions within a well-rounded program. Also, never utilize short recovery periods for high-intensity repetitions. You'll exhaust your nervous system, given that high-intensity repetitions require 2–5 minutes of nervous system recovery; short recovery periods neutralize any hoped-for gains in efficiency (running economy). Also, the energy system tapped by high-intensity repetitions requires between 1 and 3 minutes to recover. Shortening the recovery period changes the energy system you'll tap to fuel your next repetition, and that changes what muscle cells you can use. In other words, you'll no longer be training what you *think* you're training—you'll have lost control of your workout.

Mistake 5: Fast starts

When children play, they'll often transition straight from standing still to sprinting. That works for kid's games. It won't work for your running. As we discussed in Chapter 6 (page 101), when you begin your run at too fast a pace, you're forced to use an excessive amount of anaerobic energy. That leads to premature fatigue (often within minutes of starting), which results in shortened, aborted, or overly difficult workouts. You'll also be forcing muscles that haven't yet warmed up to work at an intense effort. That's a recipe for muscle strains and tendinitis.

Avoid this mistake: "Every single time we walk out the door, every single run, every single workout should be a negative split," says Sean Wade, a 1996 Olympic marathoner for New Zealand and the coach, through his Houston-based Kenyan Way running program, to more than five thousand runners who've successfully completed marathons and half marathons. "That means the first mile of a distance run should be super easy, and as we naturally warm up we should get quicker." Note that *quicker* doesn't mean fast; it means your normal distance pace.

Mistake 4: Running while injured

You feel niggling pain in your foot, shin, hammy, hip, groin, or elsewhere in your running body. Should you run? Rest? Part of you probably knows that a day off won't hurt. But another part recalls that scene from the film *Platoon* where evil Sergeant Barnes clamps his hand over the mouth of a wounded soldier and growls, "Shut up and take the pain! Take the pain!" So maybe you decide to *take the pain* and run. And the next day you can't walk without ibuprofen and a crutch.

Avoid this mistake: Pain and injury come in many different sizes and shapes. Some you can train through. Some you can't. Unfortunately, you often can't tell the difference between the two until it's too late. So if it's pain you haven't experienced before, take the day off. And then another if required. If it's a nonissue you've dealt with in the past (e.g., slightly sore calves following a hard repetition workout), then just make sure you don't overdo it. Also, remember that the absolute best way to deal with injuries is to prevent them. If you're worried about developing a particular injury, see the chart, "Identify Your Running Injury," in Chapter 12 (page 223), and then follow the injury-prevention exercises suggested.

Mistake 3: Inadequate recovery

This is another concept we've dealt with throughout this book. When you train hard, you damage muscles, bones, and tendons, deplete fuel stores and hormones, and fatigue your nervous system. Afterward, your body first repairs the damage, and then it overcompensates, creating physical adaptations that leave you fitter than before the workout. But this rebuilding takes time: two to four days after hard workouts for younger runners, and up to twice that for older runners. If you push hard every day, your body won't recover—and you'll only end up more fatigued, less fit, and back on the couch.

Avoid this mistake: "Most runners feel guilty when they take a true easy day," says Joe Rubio, a two-time Olympic Trials qualifier in the marathon and mentor for many of the USA's top distance runners as head coach of Central California's Asics Aggies. "Most fail to acknowledge that all gains in fitness are achieved during periods of recovery." Rubio believes in the hard-easy approach to training, and he also schedules one easy week per month for his runners, during which they cut their training by 20 percent. That works for his elite runners, and it will work for you, too.

BECOMING A RUNNER:
Brian Spangenberg

Brian Spangenberg, age fifty-one, of Oxnard, California, lives in a three-bedroom home (a thirty-second walk from the beach) with his mother and ten-year-old daughter, Shelby, and is an executive at Prestige Medical. Sound like a nice, normal life? Well, a few years ago, Brian was homeless, unemployed, addicted to crack, and looking at jail time. Brian hadn't started out on that path. As a high school freshman, Brian had beaten the entire track team in an early-season time trial. Coach Don Dooley had told him: "Brian, you're the difference between a champ and a chump." Proving Coach Dooley wrong, Brian quit the next day to protest a five-mile training run. Years later, in the mid-1990s, Brian tried running again. This time, he stuck with it. And by 2004 he was logging 85 to 100 miles per week. That same year, he overcame temperatures in the mid-80s to run 2:33 at the Boston Marathon, earning a top-30 finish. Things were looking up for Brian. He had a good job. Had a son, Brendan, a stepson, Dillon, and newborn daughter, Shelby. And he was touring with a rock band. "I recorded two records with a major label," he says, "but didn't make any money at that." He quit the band in 2008. And things went south in 2009. His wife, Bridget, at the suggestion of a neighbor, began using crack cocaine to relieve severe back pain. Brian joined in. "You'd think I would have gotten into trouble with the rock band," says Brian, "not with my wife." Brian was soon smoking crack every day. He got behind on bills, missed work, quit running, and descended into a self-described state of "psychosis."

Mistake 2: Monster workouts

Sixty-five million years ago, a massive asteroid collided with Earth, just off the Yucatán peninsula, and triggered a mass extinction that claimed 75 percent of animal and plant life on the planet and wiped out the dinosaurs. Monster workouts will have an analogous effect on your running

Arrested for possession, Brian couldn't find a ride home from jail. So he jogged. And found an eviction notice on his door, a termination letter from his employer, and his family gone—with his daughter and stepson soon to be taken by Children's Services (Brendan was already out of the house). When his dad died shortly thereafter, Brian says, "I had lost everything." Brian attended inpatient rehab, outpatient rehab, aftercare, separate drug and alcohol diversion classes, and countless AA and NA meetings. But his rehabilitation was stunted when he couldn't forge the connection with a "higher power," considered essential to success in his various programs. Eventually, he tried running again. The first run was hell. "The only good thing was that I was still skinny from the drugs," says Brian. He pushed on, and within a year, he raced a 10K. "Toward the end, I ran through a dark tunnel and then came out into the light," says Brian. "I thought that was symbolic." Running became his higher power. He got his job back in 2011, where he's now considered a "top executive." And got his daughter back (Dillon moved to Arizona to be with his biological father). And got back the house. And finally, miraculously, reclaimed a nice, normal, healthy, and fit lifestyle. "Running is still important," says Brian, "but the priority is family and career." Almost four decades later, Brian has finally lived up to Coach Dooley's assessment: He's a champ, not a chump.

program. A monster workout is one in which you engage in a disastrous overload of volume and intensity, based upon the false premise that if a little training is good for you, more is better. "It's a common, possibly lethal mistake to work too hard in a training session," says Tom Schwartz, who holds a master's degree in exercise science and served as a coauthor for my book *Build Your Running Body*. "As a general rule, it takes about fourteen days to recover from a super-hard workout. The consequence is no performance benefit and the possible loss of performance capacity." In other words, you do a lot of workout for nothing—and risk losing the fitness you've already achieved. While most monster workouts are pre-planned, some develop spontaneously during workouts, driven by what I call the "green-light syndrome": You increase the prescribed volume or intensity for a workout because you "feel good," believing that *feeling good* is a green light for running harder; later, you are mystified when you suddenly "feel bad" and have to take time off to recover.

Avoid this mistake: Never run a workout that is significantly more difficult than previous workouts. And never finish a workout completely exhausted. As for "green-light syndrome," remember that you're supposed to "feel good" when you're training correctly. That's the whole point! Feeling good isn't a green light for a harder workout; it's your body telling you that your training is working.

Mistake 1: Overtraining

This is the granddaddy of all training mistakes. *Overtraining* is the extended-play version of "monster workouts": Instead of body-slamming your muscles, nerves, and heart with a single Herculean effort, you spread your training gluttony over multiple days or weeks. The result is a pronounced—*and prolonged*—crash and burn. Symptoms of overtraining include impaired performance, heavy legs, muscle and joint pain, lethargy, insomnia, clumsiness, weight loss, elevated heart rate, and increased thirst at night. Overtraining syndrome can come on suddenly and then linger for six to twelve weeks, during which you'll need to reduce your training or stop altogether. Overtraining syndrome is your body's way of telling you to mellow the heck out!

Avoid this mistake: I once asked coach Jack Daniels for advice on dealing with overtraining syndrome. His answer was two words long: "Avoid it." Coach Daniels is right. And the best way to avoid it is to follow the training maxim: *Better undertrained than overtrained.* Undertrained, you can always train a little harder to chase improvement. Overtrained, it's already game over.

As a runner, you're going to make mistakes. It comes with the territory. And sometimes you'll have to pay for those mistakes—with fatigue, injuries, and, now and then, a few days off.

But here's the thing: There is no such thing as a mistake that's inevitable.

Sure, there isn't a mistake listed in this chapter that hasn't been made by countless runners in the past. And won't be made by countless more in the future.

But that doesn't mean *you* have to make it. In the next chapter, we're going to put together your personal action plan. You'll create a plan that incorporates your goals in running, scheduling, nutrition, recovery, and lifestyle. You'll be taking the concrete step of outlining the forward trajectory of your life. You don't want to mess that up with a stupid mistake.

You've probably been told more than once in this life: Learn from your mistakes.

Well, I'm here to tell you that's a no-good, rotten plan.

Instead, learn from my mistakes. And from those of all the runners who've already traveled down injury road.

Save yourself the pain, the grief, and the downtime.

CHAPTER TAKEAWAY

If you want to succeed as a runner, you must make your training a *no-mistake zone.* A single mistake can derail the most carefully constructed running plan. The first step is to identify potential mistakes. The next step is to refrain from making those mistakes by incorporating smart strategies into your program. When it comes to mistakes, it's best to learn from the experience of others—and save yourself the injuries, medical bills, and downtime on the couch.

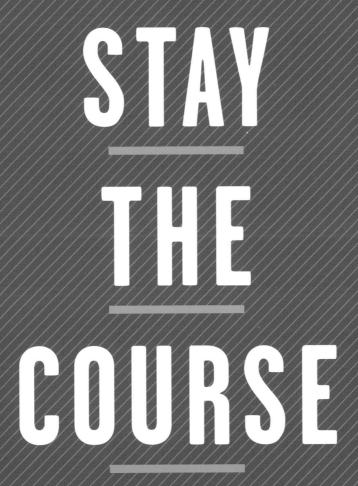

PART THREE

STAY THE COURSE

9

Create Your Personal Action Plan

"The shoe that fits one person pinches another; there is no recipe for living that suits all cases."
—CARL JUNG

OK, IT'S YOUR TURN.

It's time for me to stop telling stories, cheerleading you past obstacles, and warning you about mistakes. And time for you to take what we've discussed in this book and use it to create your personal *action plan*. Your plan will be much more than a training schedule. That's because your training schedule can only succeed when you've taken all the other elements of your life into consideration. A sustainable plan will not only account for factors such as family, work, friends, diet, time constraints, the obstacles you face, and available training facilities, it will also attend to less tangible concerns, such as the criteria you'll use to define success, the rewards you'll self-administer upon achieving goals, and the timeline you'll project for different stages of your program.

Most of you won't be able to figure out a plan like that in your head—or, even if you could, to hold it there for the months it will take to complete. So instead, you'll want to use the "Running Program Action Plan" worksheet included at the end of this chapter (page 170). The worksheet takes your big goal—*I want to run*—and breaks it into smaller, more manageable goal chunks (exercise, scheduling, diet, recovery, lifestyle, and sharing).

Then again, some of you might prefer a different medium for your plan. Maybe you want to fill in daily goals and steps on a traditional calendar. Maybe you've got a running log for entering the details of each day's workout and associated activities. Maybe you prefer simply jotting down notes on a piece of paper. Or some of you—especially experienced runners returning from injury or long breaks—might even feel that a written plan is unnecessary. You've navigated a training program in the past, and you've hardwired strategies to meet the challenge of successfully executing a new program.

And, of course, others of you might feel that this is too big a step to take right now. You're tapping all your available resources just getting out the door for a walk or a jog. You're not ready to plot out a future beyond today's workout. If that's you, don't sweat it. You can *always* come back to this chapter. For now, focus on what you *can* do.

Regardless of whether you utilize the action plan worksheet or choose a different medium (or no medium at all), you'll benefit from reading through this chapter. It will help you to think through all aspects of your coming program—imagining the person you want to become, envisioning the role that running will play in your life, and mentally navigating the path from where you stand today to where that new version of yourself awaits in the future.

For those utilizing the worksheet, we'll go step-by-step through each of its fields. If you need extra guidance in filling it out, you can refer to a completed sample action plan at bornagainrunner.com. There's also a downloadable Excel or PDF version of the action plan worksheet available at the site; if you print a hard copy of the action plan, it will be easier to fill in fields while simultaneously referencing the training schedules or other sections of this book.

It's been said that writing down goals transforms them from dreams into a plan. I'd like to amend that: Writing down goals and then outlining steps for achieving them turns dreams into an *action plan*, into a real-life blueprint for transforming your life.

YOUR RUNNING PROGRAM ACTION PLAN

The path you are about to forge is neither straight nor narrow. You cannot assume a beeline between yourself and your future running goal(s). Not unless you intend to run through (metaphorical) potholes, yellow caution tape, and brick walls. Instead, your path will navigate a terrain chockablock with commitments to family, job, friends, and your community, and also with the unforeseen—the family emergencies, the work deadlines, winter storms, a twisted ankle, the flu, a locked high school track, or any of countless situations that can spring up suddenly and disrupt your training plan.

Your action plan *must* be as versatile as the life you'll be leading. Marking down, "Run 20 minutes," on the calendar three times a week probably won't cut it. That's why the action plan worksheet includes fields under each goal for anticipating challenges and obstacles, brainstorming solutions, and developing contingency plans. Don't think of these fields as busy work. Spending a few minutes now to prepare for any and all variables will save you mountains of time (not to mention energy, anxiety, and frustration) in the future when conflicts and unexpected situations arise. Plus, a running program is such a big, amorphous beast of a concept that sometimes it's easier to break the plan into smaller pieces—and then to tackle those pieces one at a time.

The first pieces we'll be tackling are your action-plan goals. These goals embody the desired outcomes of your running program. For each of the six goals in your plan, you'll write down a general mission statement that expresses your hoped-for outcome for that goal. For example, under *exercise goal*, you might write, "Run continuously for 30 minutes, remain injury-free, and enjoy myself!" Once you've entered mission statements for each goal, you'll then determine the *action steps* you intend to take in order to achieve your goal. An action step is a specific effort, activity, or commitment. For example, again under your *exercise goal*, you might list the action step, "Begin program with 15 minutes of walking/jogging." There are lines for three action steps under each goal in this template (you can edit the downloadable Excel version of the plan), but feel free to add more lines if you need them. The six goal areas you'll be addressing are:

1 **EXERCISE GOAL:** This is where you'll identify the specific physical training (e.g., walking, running, resistance training, etc.) that you'll be including in your program, as well as any steps you'll be taking (exercise-wise) to overcome obstacles (e.g., injury-specific exercises from Chapter 12 to rehab a chronic injury). You'll probably list several steps in this section, given that you'll be altering your schedule after the first three to four weeks.

2 **DIET & NUTRITION GOAL:** Here, you'll list steps for losing weight, eating healthier, and properly fueling your training.

3 **SCHEDULING GOAL:** This is your calendar, where you'll spell out the days and time of day you intend to train, as well as listing any arrangements (e.g., child care) that will be required.

4 **RECOVERY GOAL:** You'll want to specify realistic steps for ensuring post-workout recovery and sleep.

5 **LIFESTYLE GOAL:** This section addresses your goals beyond exercise, such as eliminating bad habits (e.g., smoking), reducing stress, and expanding your social network.

6 **SHARING GOAL:** This is where you'll focus on steps to build your support team, to bring family, friends, and other runners into your running program loop.

Each of your action steps can be further defined by completing six fields in that action step's row (these fields aren't mandatory for creating a workable action plan, just recommended). These fields include:

CHALLENGES: These are the internal or external obstacles you'll face in executing the step; these can be as simple as finding a place to run or as difficult as learning how to cook healthy meals after a lifetime of frozen dinners and Pop-Tarts.

SOLUTIONS: Here, you brainstorm ways to address and overcome your challenges.

TIMELINE: You'll want to estimate (or guesstimate) when you'll be starting an action step or when you'll be finishing it (or both). Build in a little leeway, and be prepared to adjust your projections even more. Physical, mental, and lifestyle adaptations don't always follow a prepared schedule.

SUCCESS CRITERIA: You'll want to assign *success criteria* for each step. It's important for you to establish ahead of time what constitutes successful completion of a step. This helps you to visualize exactly what must be accomplished in order to complete the step. It also alerts you when it's time to move forward to a new step.

REWARD: For many steps (not all), you'll want to recognize having met your success criteria with a reward. You might promise yourself a new pair of running shoes, a celebratory dinner, a road trip to your favorite running trail, or even a slice of that chocolate pecan pie in the refrigerator—*you've earned it!*

CONTINGENCY PLAN: A contingency plan is your safety net in the event you suffer setbacks. When things go wrong, we tend to blame ourselves. We often overreact and view those setbacks as personal failures. By preplanning for bumps in the road, you'll remain in control of your program. There will be no disasters, only navigable detours.

You'll want your initial action plan to cover your first few months of running. While there's no rule against writing a plan that spans a longer period of time, it's hard to predict your health, fitness, and lifestyle changes too far out.

Now that you've got the gist of your action plan, let's look at each goal separately.

Exercise goal

Your action plan begins with your exercise goal. And remember that this is *your* goal. You aren't writing an action plan to impress someone else—so no putting down, "I want to run a marathon uphill into a headwind wearing army boots." Instead, task yourself with a goal that honestly reflects your motive for running (e.g., "Complete a 5K race!") and then write down action steps for each type of exercise you'll be scheduling. You'll need to include at least two phases of exercise: one for the first three to four weeks, when you'll focus on basic strength and conditioning, and one for the next two to three months, when you'll begin serious training. If you're rehabbing an injury or planning on limiting your exercise to non-running workouts (e.g., walking and strength training), be specific about those planned activities, too. After listing your action steps, fill in the fields that pertain to those steps. Use the sample training schedules from the middle of this book and the sample action plan from bornagainrunner.com as guides for completing this section (and remember that you can download an Excel or PDF action plan from that site, to make it easier to fill in fields while referencing the training schedules and sample plan). Some action steps and field information you'll want to consider including under this goal are:

→ Your walking and jogging plan for the first three to four weeks

→ Your walking, jogging, and running plan for the first two to three months

→ Any resistance training and injury-prevention exercises you want to include

→ Cross training activities

→ If applicable, any exercise-related steps specific to a more serious obstacle (Note: If you have a medical condition, you'll need to use the Internet links in Chapter 4 to help determine your best course of action.)

When you've finished listing your action steps, check to ensure they're sufficient to achieve your exercise goal.

Scheduling goal

Don't assume that there will be time to train. Sure, it's easy to find thirty to sixty minutes the first time you head out the door. But what about the next time? What about three times a week? Or four? Or when your workouts grow to sixty to ninety minutes? I've trained numerous athletes whose programs were derailed by an unwillingness to designate days of the week and times of day for their workouts. If you have children, you'll want to consider child care (do *not* simply assume that your significant other will happily pick up the slack). If you work long days, you'll have to train early morning, late evening, or during lunch. If weather's a problem, you'll have to craft contingency plans for when it's *too big* a problem—you'll need to investigate indoor training options or invest in outdoor solutions, such as purchasing climate-neutralizing gear. A good training schedule requires more than workouts and motivation; it requires a time and a place. Some action steps and field information you'll want to consider including under this goal are:

→ The days of the week you want to train

→ The time of day you'll train

→ The amount of time you'll require to complete your workouts

→ Target start dates for the various phases of your training (e.g., the week you'll start resistance training)

→ Day(s), time, and duration for cross training activities (if you include them)

→ Adjustments based upon weather and the availability of facilities (e.g., the hours a local high school track is open to the public)

The last thing you want to worry about when it comes to training is whether you'll even have the time or available facilities to *do* that training. You wouldn't join a gym that was closed when you wanted to work out, and you shouldn't create a training schedule that is similarly impossible to execute.

Diet & nutrition goal

If you aren't already eating a healthy diet, then you'll probably want to include some nutrition and fueling goals. If weight loss is a goal, you'll want to schedule a diet and calculate the number of calories you'll be eating each day (remember, though, that you shouldn't begin both a diet and running program on day one—see "Dieting can wait" in Chapter 2, page 23). Or, if you have a medical condition like diabetes, you might need to include stricter dietary action steps (e.g., more fiber, fewer high-sugar foods, etc.). Some action steps and field information you'll want to consider including under this goal are:

→ Improved nutrition (e.g., more fruits and vegetables, more whole grains, etc.)

→ Weight-loss goals

→ Daily calorie goals

→ Healthy food swaps (e.g., roasted seaweed snacks in place of chips)

→ Fewer visits to fast-food restaurants

→ More homemade meals (e.g., taking a sack lunch to work)

Before finalizing this part of your plan, you should read this book's Chapter 11, "Eat, Drink, and ~~Be Merry~~ Watch Your Calories." There's a lot of information on diet and nutrition that you'll want to consider.

Recovery goal

We've talked a lot about recovery. But it's not enough to pay lip service to the concept. Remember that all fitness improvements occur during recovery, not during training. So it makes no sense to create a detailed training schedule and then improvise recovery. Instead, schedule it.

Some action steps and field information you'll want to consider including under this goal are:

→ Post-workout downtime (e.g., an hour or two of relaxation)

→ Sleep (try for 7–8 hours a night)

→ A hard-easy schedule (remember that *all* days are "hard" days for your first 1–3 weeks of running)

→ Post-run carbohydrate and protein supplementation

→ Limits on non-running exercise (i.e., schedule pickup basketball, soccer, or kayaking on non-running days, and remember that those activities will impact your fatigue levels and recovery time)

If you don't schedule voluntary recovery, your body will schedule involuntary recovery—via injury, illness, and burnout. With smart planning, however, you'll recover to run another day.

Lifestyle goal

Most runners have goals beyond running performance. You want to improve your health. Or reduce your stress. Or quit drinking. Or smoking. Or watching so much bad TV. Maybe you'd like to meet other positive, active, and outgoing people. At the same time, you want to preserve the relationships you have with your family and friends. You want to stay on top of your job. You want what running has to offer, but not at the expense of the life you're already leading. In this part of your action plan, you'll address these *balance of life* issues. With careful planning, you *can* have it all. Some action steps and field information you'll want to consider including under this goal are:

→ Adjustments to work hours (e.g., you might have to adjust the hours you work in order to run while there's still daylight, or you might have to cut back on work hours)

→ Healthy living choices (e.g., you might want to quit smoking)

→ Quality time with family and friends (i.e., strategies for maintaining or increasing this time)

→ Inclusion of family and friends in your new activity (e.g., a family hike on the weekend as part of your cross training)

→ Time for non-running hobbies (e.g., you might want to slot in time for coaching your son or daughter's soccer team)

→ Time spent on nonproductive activities (e.g., you might want to cut back on the time you spend surfing the web)

→ Improving your social network (e.g., finding training partners, coaches, or running clubs)

Inevitably, your lifestyle will change at least a little (or a lot, if your goal is a life makeover). But you can control the severity of that change and guide it in a positive direction by planning ahead.

Sharing goal

This final section of your action plan is for building your support team. Some runners try to hide their new programs, afraid that failure will subject them to embarrassment or ridicule. Others hide their programs in order to make a big splash later on, imagining themselves the protagonist in a Hollywood movie: *Out of shape non-runner secretly trains and diets, then emerges to surprise former tormentors with hot bod, fast 5K, and the ability to whip up thirty-one different healthy dinners—one for each day of the month—in under ten minutes each, using nothing but a pan, olive oil, and produce from their garden!* But going it alone isn't the best way to succeed in your program. Your program isn't a two-hour movie; it's a long-term commitment that will require perseverance and consistent motivation. Letting the people in your life know about your program allows those people to offer you encouragement when you need it. That may not seem important on your first day. Or during your first week. But it will become vital if the thrill of training recedes, the weather turns bad, or your rate of improvement slows down. At that point, a support team can make the difference between success and giving your program a pink slip.

You should also consider finding a training partner. There will be days you don't want to run. Maybe it's raining. Or you had a rough day at work. Or maybe the couch, cocoa, and an episode of *Game of Thrones* is calling—*loudly*. On those days, nothing is more effective at getting your butt out the door than knowing that your training partner (or more than one) is waiting for you. If you don't have a friend who's game, approach runners at tracks, parks, or other popular running spots. Or find a local club and work out with an entire team. We also listed training partners

Samantha de la Vega

Samantha de la Vega, age fifty, was born into affluence in New York City, but her riches-to-rags story would eventually lead her to heroin addiction and a jail cell in San Francisco. It seemed that Samantha had been born under a lucky star. Her grandfather was John Hill, founder of the global public relations giant Hill + Knowlton, and her grandmother was a famous Broadway actress. With her mother and sister, Samantha lived on the ninth floor of the Dakota building at the corner of Central Park West and Seventy-second Street. But the good life ended early when Samantha, not even two years old, fell out of her apartment window, slid down a rain gutter, had her fall arrested when a nail punched through her cheekbone, and was left to dangle above the busy Manhattan streets below. Her grandfather, embarrassed by the incident, had Samantha and her sister placed in their grandmother's custody. Their grandmother promptly split up the sisters. "We had houses in the country," says Samantha, "and my grandmother would send me to live with people she'd hired to take care of [those houses]." Samantha's musical-chairs existence would include boarding schools, multiple homes, and a sense of isolation. "My best friend was a statue of Kwan Yin [the Buddhist goddess of mercy] at my grandfather's apartment. I'd talk to her, even make out with her," says Samantha. While attending a Connecticut boarding school, Samantha discovered cross country. "I loved it," she says. "I became the second runner on the team. I'd go home and be alone, but now I had and running clubs as a potential step under your *lifestyle goal*. That's because it's worth mentioning twice! If you have trouble with this step, visit the following web address to see a list of clubs in your area: usatf. org/Products---Services/Club-Memberships.aspx.

If you'd prefer virtual running friends, join the online running community. You can always find a reassuring voice and a vibrant running

something that no one could take away from me. I had my power." Unfortunately, the experience was short-lived. Only fourteen, Samantha left Connecticut for the jungles above Puerto Vallarta, Mexico, to live with her father, a well-known actor who'd renounced the material world and turned to LSD. While there, she suffered a series of mishaps and assaults. And before long, she was back in the States. At eighteen, she drifted to the San Francisco punk scene, moved in with John, a junkie, and spent eight years shooting heroin. "I thought I was being artsy and cool," she says. "I got abused, strung out, and, when I got *really* strung out, John left me." Samantha turned to dealing drugs and was arrested. She fled a diversionary drug program and moved to Mexico City. There, finally, she resurrected the activity that still resonated in her memory—and rediscovered her power. "I'd run at four in the morning, then teach English, go home, eat, and run again." She cleaned up, moved to Portland, Oregon, cleared her arrest record, and, in December 2012, finished her first ultra, the Deception Point 50K. She's completed a dozen ultras since. "Running is the thing I always come back to," says Samantha. "I leave all the sadness, and all the chaos, and I turn it into my strength, my beautiful moments."

discussion on the message boards at runnersworld.com, runningahead
.com, active.com, and other running sites.

If none of the above suggestions works for you, start a running log.
It's a place to record your runs, diet, moods, or anything else about your
running program that comes to mind. You'll be surprised at how quickly
you come to relish filling in the details of each day's run—and the pride
you'll experience looking through old entries. You can go old-school,
purchasing a running log at most brick-and-mortar bookstores (or from
online vendors). Or you can take advantage of many websites that offer
online running logs, most of them free (e.g., running-log.com and run-
ningahead.com).

Some action steps and field information you'll want to consider
including under this goal are:

→ Announcement of your goal (e.g., tell those family members,
   friends, and coworkers whom you anticipate will be supportive)

→ Online running message boards that welcome beginners or
   returning runners (e.g., community.runnersworld.com/forum/
   beginners-running)

→ A running log

→ Training partners, running clubs

There was a 1962 film (based upon a short story of the same name) titled
The Loneliness of the Long Distance Runner. Don't buy into that. For your
running journey, it's better to travel with family and friends.

Runners begin their running programs with a certain expectancy: We
will get healthier, fitter, and leaner, and we'll feel more energetic. But
that expectancy can't be fulfilled by a pair of Nikes and the one-time
motivation to charge out the door. It can only be fulfilled through careful
planning.

When you create an action plan, you aren't simply scribbling words
on paper. You're making a promise to yourself. And not the sort of half-
baked promise fueled by New Year's Eve champagne or a lonely star in

the night sky (and come on, that's not a real wishing star, anyway, it's Venus). This promise has teeth. It has detail. Heck, it has more depth, recitals, disclosures, dates, and compliance description than most legal contracts. That may not seem very exciting when you first think about it. But think again. Because I'll tell you something: Your personal action plan—far more than any vague running goal that might have been rattling around in your head—will become your inspiration as you move forward in your running program. Every time you question your ability to run, or wonder whether you'll ever accomplish your goals, or begin to think that training is robbing you of time better spent on some other activity, you'll look at your action plan—at your crystal ball into your fitness and lifestyle future—and you'll see that everything, absolutely everything, is going according to plan.

CHAPTER TAKEAWAY

You'll need more than a training schedule to create a sustainable running program. You'll need to create an action plan that accounts for all the factors in your life that affect your program: your family, career, diet, hobbies, and other non-running activities and considerations. An action plan breaks your overall running program goal into a half dozen smaller goals, then anticipates obstacles associated with those goals, brainstorms solutions, and offers contingency plans when things go awry. While an action plan may seem like a lot of work, it will save you time and frustration in the long run. Plus, it's one of the best ways to ensure success in your running program goals.

Running Program Action Plan

Exercise Goal

Action	Steps	Challenges	Solutions	Timeline
1				
2				
3				

Scheduling Goal

Action	Steps	Challenges	Solutions	Timeline
1				
2				
3				

Diet & Nutrition Goal

Action	Steps	Challenges	Solutions	Timeline
1				
2				
3				

Recovery Goal

Action	Steps	Challenges	Solutions	Timeline
1				
2				
3				

Lifestyle Goal

Action	Steps	Challenges	Solutions	Timeline
1				
2				
3				

Sharing Goal

Action	Steps	Challenges	Solutions	Timeline
1				
2				
3				

Success Criteria   Rewards   Contingency Plan

Success Criteria   Rewards   Contingency Plan

Success Criteria   Rewards   Contingency Plan

Success Criteria   Rewards   Contingency Plan

Success Criteria   Rewards   Contingency Plan

Success Criteria   Rewards   Contingency Plan

10

Live the Running Life

"It is better to travel well than to arrive."

—BUDDHA

FOR MANY OF YOU, creating your running program action plan is akin to a teenager getting handed the keys to the car. You're ready to go. Now. You took driver's ed. Passed your driver's test. Received your license. You're ready to put the rubber to the road. Except that you're not ready yet.

Because you haven't yet learned the rules of the road.

Sure, you've watched runners scuttle back and forth on roads, trails, and sidewalks, like ants scouting food for the colony, but there's actually a bit more to it than that. For one thing, there's runner's etiquette, a way of interacting with runners and non-runners alike (e.g., walkers, bikers, and cars) that ensures peaceful coexistence. And there are safety practices that will help get you home in one piece. And tips to prevent you from getting lost, running the wrong way on the track, or getting stranded in the Porta-Potty line a few minutes before your 5K race. You'll need to know the simple things—like where to run and, more importantly, where *not* to run;

and what to do when nature calls five miles into a ten-mile run; and how to defend yourself when a dog snaps at your heels. You'll need to know all the various customs, protocols, tricks, and behaviors that we runners utilize on a daily basis to practice our sport in the most efficient, safe, and considerate manner possible. You'll need to know how to live the running life.

FIRST THINGS FIRST: *WHERE CAN I RUN?*

Of course, the first thing you'll need to know as a runner—and something we've touched on in past chapters—is where, in fact, you can run. The answer is pretty much this: Anywhere, as long as you observe the specific rules for that running venue. Some options include:

PUBLIC ROADS: Most public roads allow runners to use shoulders and sidewalks. But since there are roads that don't—the interstate comes to mind—check local laws.

GRASSY MERIDIANS: Runners often train on the grassy center meridians of roads. If you do (and if it's legal where you live), make sure to obey all stoplights at intersections.

PUBLIC TRAILS: A sign at the trailhead will usually indicate if you're allowed access. You'll also learn whether horses and cyclists will be sharing the trail.

PUBLIC PARKS: Most parks post signs letting you know what is and isn't allowed. That said, most public parks allow running. Just be courteous to others using the park and never run through picnics or organized events.

LOCAL HIGH SCHOOL AND COLLEGE TRACKS: Most tracks post the hours that they're open for public use—*if* they allow public use. Also, school sports teams always get priority.

THE RULES OF THE ROAD (AND TRAIL)

When you run on public roads and trails, you should be aware of both the laws governing pedestrians and the unwritten safety guidelines practiced by most runners. While the two are often synonymous, the reality is that there are occasions where you'll bend the law in order to observe the prime directive of your runs: *Make it home safely.*

Run against traffic

This is the law. Legally, you should run on the side of the road (your left-hand side in the USA) that positions you to face oncoming traffic. The idea is that you'll see a car approaching dangerously close to you and be able to leap to safety. Now for the reality: You are *just as likely* to get hit by a car coming toward you as you are by one approaching from behind. And when you run facing the traffic, your odds of getting hit by cars entering the roadway from driveways or side streets increases dramatically—that's because drivers entering a roadway often look *only* in the direction of oncoming traffic, which is the opposite direction from you. That means they won't see you, and, especially if they're in a hurry, they might not stop for you.

RUNNER STRATEGY: Obey the law when you can. Very few runners get hit by cars, so your risk is minimal no matter which direction you face. On blind curves—because drivers tend to hug these curves, drifting into the shoulder area where you're running—hold your arm away from your body; drivers will steer toward your extended hand, not your torso. If there are lots of driveways and side streets, run on the sidewalk going in the same direction as traffic (that way drivers entering the roadway will look in your direction before merging, and you won't be breaking the law by running the "wrong way" on the road).

Stay on sidewalks or the shoulder of the road

In other words, stay out of the middle of the road. The road is for cars. Sidewalks are safest, but many runners feel that the combination of cement (which is harder than asphalt) and numerous dips for driveways and curbs leads to increased post-run stiffness. (Since we've raised the issue of surface hardness, most runners do best splitting their runs between roads and trails—the roads create more impact force on your legs, but the softer trails lead to "wobbling" over the uneven terrain, which contributes to connective tissue injuries.) If you're on the road, hug the outside of the shoulder, leaving as much space as possible between you and vehicles on the road. Bike lanes are great, but bikers don't like sharing—also, if there is an adjacent sidewalk or shoulder, you just might be breaking the law by using the bike lane.

Stop at intersections

Always. Stop whether the intersection has a stoplight, a stop sign, or no controlled stoppage at all. Even if you have a green light. Even if it's in the middle of the night and no one else is on the highway. Pause before crossing. More than 50 percent of serious runner-vehicle accidents occur at intersections. If you get a red light, stop; wait for a green light and the WALK sign. Jog in place if you want (although your legs won't stop working if you don't). Once, when I was fourteen years old, I tried to outrace the flashing DON'T WALK signal. I lost. And got clipped by a car accelerating into a left-hand turn. I rolled over the hood and windshield, then was tossed into the street, bloody and bruised—a small price to pay if I can convince you to act otherwise.

Jaywalk at your own risk

All runners jaywalk. We cross roads where it's not allowed—to sidestep roadwork, to detour around dogs, or to avoid the worst-of-the-worst blind curves (sometimes they're just *too* dangerous). Two things. One, don't do it if you don't have to—it's risky and gives runners a bad rap when drivers have to brake. Two, only do it if you're certain you've got a clear path and plenty of time to make it across; I've witnessed runners and pedestrians misjudge both, once with a lethal outcome (I'll never forget that, and I don't want *you* to forget this advice, either).

Run on the right, pass on the left

On sidewalks and trails, run on the right-hand side and pass on the left-hand side. Also, when you're passing someone, let them know ahead of time that you're coming (e.g., "Jogger on your left!"). And, yes, when you're certain you have that stretch of sidewalk or trail all to yourself, it's OK to ignore this rule and run in the middle or on the left-hand side.

Finally, don't overreact when other runners don't follow this rule. They might not know the rule. And, regardless, it's not worth a battle. You're running. Not claiming territory.

Drivers aren't the boss of you

Drivers will sometimes wave you across roads or intersections (in front of their cars) when you clearly don't have the right-of-way. Ignore them. Yes, they're trying to be polite. But they also might get you hurt. They can't control what the driver behind them will do, and that driver might get impatient, swing wide, speed around the stopped car, and plow straight into you. Also, it's illegal, and chances are the driver will be long gone by the time the police officer finishes writing your citation. Just wave a *thanks* and decline the right-of-way. Never surrender control of your run or safety.

No littering, pooping, or peeing on private property

You'll soon discover that there are far fewer garbage cans and restroom facilities in the great outdoors than you previously suspected. If you're holding on to litter (e.g., an empty gel pack), keep holding on to it until you find a garbage can. If nature calls, you might not have that luxury. But desperation is no excuse for making someone's yard your bathroom. Instead, you'll need to plan ahead for just this type of situation.

RUNNER STRATEGY: First, plot a running route that takes you near as many public restrooms as possible (evenly distributed throughout the route). Second, anticipate trouble by using the bathroom before you run. Third, run on a mostly empty stomach (unless this isn't an issue for you). Fourth, stop and walk when the urge becomes overpowering—the sensation sometimes eases up when you're not running. Fifth, if you absolutely can't make it to a restroom, find a clump of bushes that conceals you completely from passersby (some runners carry toilet paper for just such occasions).

Going exploring

One of the best parts of running is exploration. It's a rush to explore a new trail, climb a new mountain, or play tourist in a new city—or to plan a vacation around all three. On the other hand, it's a major bummer to get lost while doing any of that. Here are some tips for keeping your bearings:

→ Leave your expected itinerary (no matter how vague) with someone, and let them know how long you expect to be gone.

→ Carry the address of your start point, so that you can ask for directions.

→ Carry a phone with GPS mapping (make sure it's completely charged). If you get lost, it will steer you back to your start point. Or you can call someone for assistance.

→ Limit the number of turns you make during a run. This applies to both roads and trails. On the roads, you'll have a hard time remembering more than a handful of street names (especially if you get fatigued). On the trails, consider always going "right" or always going "left" at forks—that way, you can do the opposite on the return to retrace your steps. Routes look *very* different when run from different directions, so don't trust your visual memory.

→ And the best tip: Run with a local who knows the way.

Safety first

To end this section, let's review a quick bullet-point list on safety. Yes, you've heard some of this before. No, that doesn't mean you shouldn't read it again.

→ When you run at night, wear reflective clothing—or at least choose visible colors like red and white for your outfits.

→ If you're wearing headphones, keep the volume low (one earbud out is best) so that you can hear cars, cyclists, other runners, and strangers making a surreptitious approach.

→ When you run alone, take precautions. Let someone else know where you're going and how long you expect to be gone. Carry identification. If approached by anyone who makes you feel ill at ease, find another adult, approach them, and explain the situation—if no one is around, flag down a car.

→ Never cross in front of a car that's stopped at a stop sign, traffic signal, driveway, side street, or otherwise until you've made eye contact with the driver. Never assume that the driver has seen you.

→ If the driver of a car wants the right-of-way, regardless of whether it's yours, in spite of the fact that the law is on your side, *give the car the right-of-way.* In the battle of car versus human, the car always wins.

→ On trails, give mountain bikes the right-of-way. It's more dangerous for the mountain biker than for you in that situation. That's because it's harder for bike riders to stop or maneuver. Plus, a quick break won't affect your run one bit, and you just might get a hearty "Thank you!" as a reward. Meaning you'll get to feel good about yourself for the next few miles.

THE ANIMAL KINGDOM

Where I live, coyotes, mountain lions, horses, and snakes are all part of the scenery. Especially coyotes. When I was a kid, the coyotes were scraggly and underfed, and they bolted every time they caught sight of a human. Nowadays, they're the size of small German shepherds, boast glossy coats, and are fearless. A few years ago, I was jogging on a remote trail, and I noticed a coyote pacing me on the hillside to my left. I didn't think much of it until I heard scrambling in the brush to my right—and noticed a coyote pacing me on that side, too. I made some noise, and they broke off their hunt. But it was a reminder that we runners need to stay aware of our surroundings. Sure, you may not meet coyotes or mountain lions, but you'll most likely have to deal with dogs at some point. Or maybe bees. Possibly birds. Mind you, almost all of your interspecies run-ins will be peaceful. But it pays to be prepared.

DOGS OFF-LEASH (OWNER PRESENT): I've yet to be bitten by a dog whose owner didn't immediately proclaim, "My dog doesn't bite." And I've been bitten a half dozen times. One dog exited a driveway one hundred yards up a side street, raced down the street, dodged traffic across a busy road, and then sunk its teeth into my Achilles tendon. The owner explained, "You did something to antagonize him." I love dogs. I'm a dog owner. But understand that dogs bite. Even nice dogs. Runners can trigger an instinctive chase response in some dogs that walkers won't. Dog owners don't always understand this. *Fido doesn't bite me,* they think, *and he doesn't bite family and friends*; ipso facto, *Fido won't bite a runner.* Until Fido does. Bottom line: Always stop running when you encounter a dog that's off-leash. Walk past the dog. Insist that the owner call the dog—don't ask, tell (i.e., "Call your dog!"). Don't be rude. Just firm. It's probably a really nice dog. But that won't make its bite hurt any less.

DOGS OFF-LEASH (NO OWNER PRESENT): If a dog approaches you aggressively during a run, *don't* run from it. That will only increase the likelihood that it will chase and possibly bite you. Instead, stop. If the dog remains aggressive, tell it, "No!" If that doesn't do it, either pick up a rock or pretend to pick one up. Don't throw the rock (it's not the dog's fault that its owner is irresponsible); just imply that you might—that's usually enough to keep the dog at bay. Walk away slowly, keeping your eye on the dog, until you've exited its territory.

DOGS ON A LEASH: Don't assume the dog is safe. Give it a wide berth. Even when on a leash, dogs will sometimes lunge at runners. If you're on a narrow sidewalk or trail and can't put a leash's distance between you and the dog, then walk. As Ronald Reagan opined on his dealings with the Soviet Union, "Trust, but verify."

HORSES: Horses get nervous around runners. So do horse riders. On narrow trails, always stop and walk past a horse. If you're approaching the horse from behind, call out from at least fifty feet away, "Jogger approaching." (Note: The word *jogger* elicits a less-startled reaction from people than the word *runner.*) Then slow down. And walk past the horse (if the rider refuses to adjust the horse's pace so that this is possible, then jog slowly). A horse can be a danger to both you and its rider. Yes, it will break up your run to walk, but that's better than a kick in the face.

SNAKES: I remember the first time I saw a rattlesnake go from stretched out across a trail to coiled and ready to strike. It took a fraction of a second. If you see a snake, give it a wide berth. Don't jump over it. If you don't see the snake until you're about to step on it, do what you can (twist and turn) to miss it—then get the heck away.

BEES: If you see a sign warning you that there are bees in the area, believe it. Bees will sting if they think you're a threat to their hive. This doesn't mean you should panic whenever you see a bee. You shouldn't. Just exercise caution when there's a hive nearby. And if a bee lands on you, don't swat it; brush it away gently or simply exercise patience—eventually, it'll fly away. If you're part of the 3 percent of people who are severely allergic to bee stings, ask your doctor if you should carry an epinephrine autoinjector on your run.

BIRDS: Like bees, birds will sometimes become aggressive when defending their nests or territory. Dive-bombing owls, red-winged blackbirds, seagulls, mockingbirds, hawks, and others have been documented. Short of wearing a helmet, your best bet is to avoid areas where attacks have been reported; you'll need to wait out the nesting season that usually precipitates such behavior. It's illegal to harass or injure the birds. Ditto on moving or destroying their nests. Some birds are reluctant to swoop when you can see them, so (I'm serious) you might consider drawing or printing out a large pair of eyes, then taping them to the back of a hat, which you then wear while running. Another word of warning: Attacks aren't limited to the air. Geese—don't laugh, geese can be *nasty*—might try to run you down, nipping at your posterior with powerful beaks.

COYOTES: Attacks are infrequent, but, even so, remember that coyotes aren't pets. If you see a coyote, don't panic. You're bigger than it is; the coyote knows that. If the coyote no longer has the element of surprise, it almost certainly won't follow or otherwise bother you.

MOUNTAIN LIONS AND BOBCATS: If you live in an area with either of these, don't run alone in places where they've been spotted. If you see one, head in the opposite direction. If you see a baby, don't linger and sigh, "It's so cute!" It's got a mother nearby, and mom won't like you messing with her cub.

BEARS: Ditto on all of the above. If you *do* encounter a bear, you'll want to make some noise and wave your arms—that way it'll know you're a human. Don't run away; back away. If you run regularly in bear country, try to avoid dawn and dusk (when bears are most active), avoid salmon streams and areas with lots of berries, stay alert (no headphones), and consider carrying some EPA-approved bear pepper spray. Also, if you run with a dog, keep Fido on a leash to prevent Fido from annoying the bear.

CROCODILES AND ALLIGATORS: Do we really have to even discuss this?

OTHER ANIMALS (E.G., RACCOONS, DEER, SKUNKS, SQUIRRELS, AND, FOR THOSE OF YOU IN THE PACIFIC NORTHWEST, BIG-FOOT): Use your best judgment. Remember that our fellow species don't run for sport. If you're running, they figure you're either predator or prey.

TRAINING WITH PARTNERS AND GROUPS

The basic rules of the road (and trail) remain the same for outings with training partners and groups. But you'll want to know more than basic rules. You'll want to bone up on your runner-to-runner etiquette—that is, if you want to get invited back. You'll also want to exercise a little fore-sight in picking your running mates; a long run can become a *really* long run with the wrong partners.

Choosing your training partners or running group

You should consider the following five factors when choosing training partners, a training group, or a running club:

FITNESS: You'll want training partners who are running approximately the same pace and distance for their workouts as you are. Running with people who are faster than you won't get you fit faster; it will burn you out. Ditto for going farther than your fitness dictates.

GEOGRAPHY: Your training partners should be local. First, it will take less travel time to meet them for workouts. Second, if anyone cancels at the last minute, no one else gets stuck having driven an hour to train alone.

MOTIVATION & GOALS: If you're all working toward a similar goal (e.g., weight loss, overall fitness, or a fall marathon), you'll provide support and motivation for one another.

SCHEDULE: Training with other people only works if your schedules (the times you can train) are compatible. You can't run with someone who's working during the only time you have free.

PERSONALITY: Look, you're going to spend a lot of one-on-one time with your training partner(s). There isn't much to do on a run but chat (you can't always be breathless, charging up a hill). If you don't like each other, you won't like running together.

If you're having a tough time finding running partners, you should consider some of the apps available for accomplishing just that: PacePal (pacepal.com) and Jaha (jaha.com) will get you started.

Group running etiquette

When you're running with a group, you'll need to be aware of the rules governing your group's interaction with all others on the roads and trails, and you'll want to be aware of general guidelines for interacting with others in the group. Let's start with etiquette pertaining to the group as a whole:

→ You're a group, not a gang. Be respectful of others on the roads and trails—that means walkers, cyclists, horseback riders, drivers, or anyone using the same space.

→ Groups should run either single-file or two-abreast on busy roads and sidewalks; make room for others.

→ Make sure everyone in the group knows the route before you start a run. It takes less time to give directions than it does to find someone who's lost.

→ Pace should be set by what works best for the group as a whole—*not* by what works best for the fastest runner in the group.

→ Never start a run early (i.e., prior to the scheduled start time) unless everyone is already present.

Next, let's look at your responsibilities to the group:

BE ON TIME: It's hard enough to block out one or more times a week when the entire group can meet. If you're late on a regular basis, expect to find the group already on a run when you arrive late again.

ONE-STEPPING: "One-stepping" is our sport's term for a runner who insists on staying a half step or full step ahead of everyone else in the group. It's annoying, and it disrupts the group's pace (as other runners try to close the gap). It's a run, not a race.

GPS UPDATES: If runners want to know how far or how fast they've run, they'll ask. Regular updates (e.g., "We did that mile in 8:35 pace . . . Now we're at 8:27 . . .") are not appreciated by runners just trying to get their Zen on.

SELFIES: Don't initiate multiple stops for selfies without discussing it with the group first.

BREATHLESS CONVERSATION: If someone is really sucking air, maybe save the conversation with him or her for later.

ENDLESS CONVERSATION: It's a group run, not a group audience. If you absolutely must recount every single gripping moment of your week, at least save it for coffee afterward and pick up the bill.

PASSING GAS: Everyone does this on runs. That said, if you're experiencing unusually frequent backfires, consider bringing up the rear for that particular run.

ROUND AND ROUND (TRACK ETIQUETTE)

Many runners prefer training at their local track. It's safe. The footing is always good. Many tracks have lights for night training. You always know exactly how far you're running (unless you lose count of laps). And there's a built-in feeling of community with the other runners and walkers. To make sure you're always welcome at the track, here are some general guidelines:

GEAR: Stow your gear off the track (i.e., keep it out of the running lanes). Also, don't leave gear on the turf if football, soccer, or some other sport is using the field. There's usually space adjacent the outside lane (especially near the start line) for gear.

RUN COUNTERCLOCKWISE: For most of your walking and running, you'll want to go counterclockwise. If you're using the inside three lanes, you *must* run counterclockwise.

WARM-UP: Use the outside lanes (4 through 8 on most tracks) for warming up and slower running. While most runners go counterclockwise during warm-ups, some runners (especially highly competitive or high-volume runners) prefer clockwise. If you run clockwise, give way to runners going counterclockwise.

FAST RUNNING: The inside lanes are usually reserved for faster running, such as repetitions (although this rule isn't always enforced). If you see runners doing speed work or repetitions, leave the inside lanes free for them. If you're doing repetitions using the inside lanes, move to the outside lanes during your recovery interval (jog) between repetitions.

DISTANCE RUNNING: If you're doing distance runs on the track, you can use the inside lanes if they're open. While tracks are four laps to a mile (actually 1600 meters, but close enough), many tracks will list the total distance covered when running in other lanes; for example, in lane eight, it's three and a half laps for one mile (seven laps for two miles).

NON-RUNNERS IN LANES 1 TO 3: If walkers or joggers are using the inside lanes when you're attempting to do faster training, ask them politely to move to the outside lanes. I've rarely run across people who won't happily comply; they aren't being rude, they just don't understand the rules. If they won't move, don't sweat it. Just run around them (and, no, don't cut it close just to give them a scare). I tell my competitive athletes that this is good practice for racing.

TWO OR THREE ABREAST: While it's fun to spread across the lanes with your walking or running partners, it's rude to everyone else using the track. If your group is taking up more than one lane (and if others are using the track), you need a new formation.

BE A GOOD GUEST: You are an ambassador for all runners when you're on a track. If a school official or coach asks you to switch lanes or train at a different time, do it. Recognize that school teams have priority for using the facility; team training times are often posted at the entrance gate. That said, it's perfectly OK to ask a coach if you can train at the same time that his or her team is practicing. A little respect and politeness will go a long way to maintaining your access to a track.

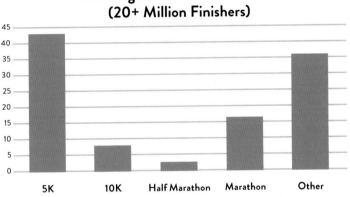

Percentage of 2015 Race Finishers (20+ Million Finishers)

RACE TIPS & ETIQUETTE

If you decide to race—whether for completion or competition—the experience should be a highlight of your running program. Most pre-race anxiety and during-race confusion (factors that sometimes spoil the experience) can be traced to a lack of information. Let's correct that.

Pre-race

The first thing you'll want to do is preregister for your race. Up until a day or two before the race, you can usually do this online through the official race website. This will save you time the morning of the race. Lines for day-of-event registration can be long. If you've preregistered, there will be lines at the registration tables based upon either the first letter of your last name or a number that's been assigned to you—if this number wasn't emailed or snail-mailed to you, it'll be printed out on a nearby poster or will be available via printed sheets on a table adjacent the registration area. Some other things to keep in mind pre-race:

ARRIVE EARLY: Traffic congestion increases and available parking decreases as race time draws near.

PARKING: Check the race website for a map of available parking. You'll want to know exactly where to park in advance.

BRING ID: You'll probably need to show identification to receive your race bib and race chip (if the race is using timing chips).

RACE BIB: This is a square or rectangular printed number that you'll attach to the front of your race shirt. Use four safety pins to make sure your bib doesn't flap around during the race. Position your bib in the center of your shirt; race photographers will sort your photos afterward with this number. Also, if your race chip malfunctions, race officials will use your bib number to spot you at the finish line or to spot you at timing mats for longer races (like marathons) in order to assign you correct finish and split times.

RACE CHIPS: Race chips help the race timing company to electronically record your finish time (and split times along the course). Chips come in several forms (e.g., tiny squares that you attach to your shoes via plastic twisties, plastic swirls that you'll thread through your laces, or transponder chips already embedded in your race bib). Some chips are disposable, and some will be collected in the finish area (if the latter, there will be race volunteers available to help you remove them). Race chips communicate with start mats, timing mats throughout the race, and finish mats. With chips, your race time doesn't start with the horn (or gun); it starts when you physically cross the start mat—and stops when you cross the finish mat.

PORTA-POTTIES: Almost all races provide Porta-Potties near the start area (and along the course). Use them early (e.g., thirty to sixty minutes before your race), as lines can get *very* long near the race start time.

LINING UP: You'll line up at the start line based upon expected pace.

The fastest runners line up at the front, with slower runners toward the middle or back of the field. Many races assign "corrals" based upon expected pace (you'll write this pace on your entry form). Races will also have pace signs (usually expressed as pace per mile) posted at various intervals in the start field. Find a position that best represents your expected pace. With chips, you won't add seconds (or minutes) to your finish time no matter how long it takes you to cross the start line.

The race

A running race is a unique event in the sporting world. It's one of the very few events where athletes of every ability compete together. New runners and Olympians line up side by side. There can be as few as a couple dozen and as many as fifty thousand participants toeing the line. So it's understandable that you might experience a case of nerves. Toward that end, here's a little of what you can expect—and what you should consider doing.

START LINE: Be prepared for a wait at the start line. All those dozens or thousands of runners have to find a place in the start field. Then there'll be a rendering of "The Star Spangled Banner." And then there will be obligatory race instructions and a speech or two from local luminaries (e.g., race sponsors or the mayor). Don't talk over the speakers. If you get frustrated with the wait—*don't*. It won't quicken the pace, and it will only escalate your anxiety levels for the actual race.

THE START: Don't start running until the person in front of you has started running. Even then, take small strides and be careful not to step on anyone. Once you start running, don't suddenly stop. There are hundreds (thousands) of runners behind you, and someone will step on you—and then you'll both go down. If you drop something, leave it; you'll get trampled reaching for it.

ON THE COURSE: Don't swerve back and forth. Runners behind you are focused on their own races and might not anticipate your movement (a recipe for a runner pileup). If the course has turns (and it will), run "tangents"—the shortest distance between you and the turn ahead is a straight line to that turn. There will be mile markers along the way if you don't have a GPS watch. And there will be aid stations to provide water and sometimes energy drinks (e.g., Gatorade) at regular intervals.

RACE MANEUVERS: If someone passes you, stay right. Never block another runner. Not only is it rude, it's against the rules.

BECOMING A RUNNER: *Suzanne Rybak*

Suzanne Rybak, age fifty-two, of Thousand Oaks, California, had her hands full with three children (Caroline, Jackson, and Will), her husband, and a black Labrador puppy when she started running a decade ago—her first serious attempt to commit to a structured exercise program. Growing up, fitness hadn't been a consideration. "I was a total bookworm and introvert," she says. "We didn't even have a track or cross country team at St. Joseph High School." It was the Labrador puppy who changed everything. After dropping her youngest off at preschool, Suzanne would train the puppy, including walks. By the end of the walks, she'd surrender to the puppy's tugging and break into some gentle running. And, in the process, she got her first taste of the endorphin rush that hooks so many runners. "I started to leave the dog home for a short two or three miles," she says, "and then come back and get it." As Suzanne's interest in running increased, the trick was finding the time to do it. "Once [the kids] were off school, there were multiple activities to do. So, initially, I ran after I dropped everybody off at school." She found it was a great way to clear her head and get organized for the day. Plus, she discovered she had more energy for the remainder of the day. When her friend Susan, a former competitive cyclist, suggested they train together, the workouts were moved to 5 AM to accommodate Susan's work schedule. "I thought there was no way I was going to run in the dark with a headlamp," Suzanne says, "but somehow I caught

UNTIED SHOE: If your shoe comes untied, move to the side of the road (or a sidewalk)—out of the way of other runners—before stopping to tie it.

TRAFFIC: Yield to emergency vehicles, police vehicles, and wheelchair athletes. Also, yield to regular vehicular traffic if there's no one there to

the bug." The two training partners would hit the roads three or four times a week, incorporating speed work and higher mileage. Before long, they decided to target a marathon. And while Susan got sidelined, Suzanne completed the Long Beach Marathon (Long Beach, California). "All my training paid off," says Suzanne. "I was just hungry for more." But those runs had prepared Suzanne for more than marathoning. "When you're training for a marathon with your girlfriends," she says, "it's the perfect opportunity to vent and get feedback—to think a little bit more deeply about where I might be going, to contemplate the future." Suzanne realized that she was unhappy in her marriage, and she filed for divorce. "Running was the one thing I had every day that made me feel empowered and peaceful about my decision." Three years later, now an apparel buyer for Future Track Running Center, Suzanne still relies on running to sort out her day. "Every morning, it's my prayer. It sets the tone for my day. When I wake up and feel like I've got way too much on my plate, I hit the road and do my six to eight miles. And it settles me. It washes away any fears I had about not being able to handle my responsibilities."

handle traffic control—there should be, but if there's not, remember the rule we discussed previously: In car versus runner, car wins.

POTTY BREAK: If you need to visit a restroom, locate an available Porta-Potty on the course. If you can't find one, ask a homeowner or stop at an open restaurant or retail business. Be polite and accept "no" for an answer. As a last resort (and only then!), use a clump of bushes and make sure no other race competitors or spectators can see you.

OTHER BODILY FUNCTIONS: If you have to spit, blow your nose, or vomit, be careful not to do it on your fellow racers. Move off the course, then do your thing.

DON'T CHEAT: It pains me to put this on the list. But I've learned (the hard way) that runners *will* cheat. I want to make sure that you don't accidentally go that route. So here we go: no cutting the course; no starting early and waiting for the field to catch you; no taking a car, bus, or cab for part of the race; no switching bibs and (or) race chips with someone younger and faster than you; and no performance-enhancing drugs. The only way you *won't* cross the finish line a winner is if you cross the finish line a cheater.

For more information on running and race etiquette, as well as on races in general, visit the Road Runners Club of America at rrca.org.

The laws, rules, customs, precautions, tricks, and tips we've covered in this chapter may seem like a lot to grasp—especially when you're still trying to absorb the training advice covered in the preceding chapters—but I think you'll find that, in practice, a lot of what we've discussed is simply common sense (and common courtesy). The reality is that you can begin your first run without committing a single item from this chapter to memory. But the reality is also that your runs, running relationships, and running safety will improve as your understanding of the sport's culture improves. Immerse yourself in that culture, and you'll soon be joining the millions of runners who are already living the running life.

CHAPTER TAKEAWAY

While it might seem like there isn't much to the act of running on sidewalks, roads, trails, and tracks, there is actually a well-defined set of laws, customs, and protocols that guides the behavior of runners. There's established etiquette for interactions between runners and other runners—and also for interactions with cyclists, horses, cars, and others. There are safety precautions. And laws (e.g., facing traffic when running). And rules (e.g., running counterclockwise on a track). And there is a multitude of tips and tricks for navigating your way through each workout in the most proficient, safe, and rewarding way possible. Absorbing all of this is your ticket to living the running life.

11

Eat, Drink, and ~~Be Merry~~ *WATCH YOUR CALORIES*

> *"The man who counts the bits of food*
> *he swallows is never satisfied."*
> —AFRICAN PROVERB

THIS ISN'T A DIET OR RECIPE BOOK. I'm not much of a cook. And I've spent most of my running life surviving on meals cobbled together from cereal, dairy products, bananas, energy bars, canned foods, pasta, and items plucked straight from the frozen-foods section of the supermarket. But that doesn't mean that I haven't made proper nutrition a central pillar of my training program. I wouldn't think of running on a diet that contained less than the required carbohydrates, protein, fat, vitamins, and minerals I need to fuel my training and strengthen my body.

Yes, it's true that your diet alone won't initiate running fitness. You can't consume a head of lettuce or a whole wheat bagel and expect to trigger the physiological changes that transform your running body—training does that. But no, that doesn't mean diet isn't important. Those physiological changes are only possible when your body receives the nutrition it requires to repair and rebuild itself. And if you're looking to lose weight, it becomes doubly important that the calories you eat provide the nutrition your body craves.

In this chapter, we'll take a look at the basic requirements for a runner's diet. We'll look at your diet from an energy standpoint—the types of fuel your body needs to train, how much you need, and where to get it. We'll find out why proteins have been called the "building blocks of life." We'll look at fat's role in preventing injuries. We'll create a list of vitamins and minerals you'll need to succeed. And, of course, we'll have a discussion about going on a diet—how to determine a healthy weight-loss goal, and then how to achieve it.

WHAT A RUNNER'S BODY NEEDS

The first thing your body needs, when it comes to food, is enough of it. Enough carbohydrates. Enough protein. Enough fat. And enough vitamins and minerals. But "enough" isn't determined by lumping together all the food you eat as one big mound of "calories." That'd be like taking all the running you do—the distance, repetitions, tempo, sprints, and races—and lumping it together as "mileage." A dietary calorie (like a mile or a kilometer) is simply a unit of measurement; technically, it represents the amount of energy it takes to raise the temperature of one kilogram of water by one degree. While there will be time for calorie counting later in this chapter, that shouldn't be your primary concern when devising your running diet. Your primary concern should center on getting the necessary amount of each macronutrient (carbs, proteins, and fats), vitamin, and mineral you'll need to build your new, fitter, healthier body.

Carbohydrates

Carbohydrates are one of the two main sources of energy for your training. Carbs are found in a wide variety of foods, including pasta, fruit, beans, popcorn, potatoes, vegetables, cookies, pie, dairy products, and pretty much everything else that isn't straight protein or fat.

Carbohydrates are stored within your muscle cells as muscle *glycogen*. Don't let the term *glycogen* confuse you—glycogen is just a form of carbohydrate, like an apple is a type of fruit, and it's the major source of carbohydrate energy you'll use while running. Every single one of your muscle cells has its own glycogen fuel tank, a tank that no other muscle cell can access. If those glycogen tanks are relatively full at the beginning of a run, you'll feel good on your run. If they're low or empty, however, you'll feel fatigued and sluggish from the start.

An average person stores 1,200 to 1,600 calories of glycogen within his or her muscles. You begin to deplete that glycogen as soon as you start exercising. If you're walking, about 17 percent of the calories you burn will come from glycogen. As you increase your pace, you also increase the percentage of calories from glycogen—to almost 50 percent for regular distance runs and 100 percent by the time you reach one-mile race pace. If you have full glycogen tanks, none of these workouts should be a problem. But if your tanks are low, you risk *bonking*, which is a term used to describe the sudden onset of extreme fatigue. In marathons, runners sometimes describe "hitting the wall" when their muscle glycogen stores get extremely low, usually around the 20-mile mark.

The takeaway for you: Always keep your muscle glycogen tanks topped off to ensure more energetic and enjoyable running. The best way to keep those tanks full is to eat plenty of carbs. The Academy of Nutrition and Dietetics recommends that endurance athletes (that's you) get between 2.3 and 5.5 grams of carbohydrates per pound of body weight. So, for example, if you weigh 150 pounds, you'll need a minimum of 345 grams of carbohydrates per day (because 2.3 x 150 = 345). And remember that you should consume a carbohydrate supplement immediately post-exercise, when your body replaces glycogen stores at an accelerated rate.

Fats

Fats are your body's second major source of energy for running. Packing nine calories per gram (versus four calories for both carbs and protein), fat is your body's most concentrated source of energy. And, as you might have noticed, it tastes pretty good, too. Our craving for fat is thought to result from evolution. After all, it made sense to load up on fat, with its high-density energy, back when our persistence-hunting ancestor, *Australopithecus*, faced the constant threat of food scarcity. These days, however, with fatty products crowding the supermarket shelves, overindulgence has helped create a worldwide health issue. There are more than 1.5 billion overweight adults on the planet (half a billion of them characterized as obese), leading to 2.8 million deaths per year.

Of course, you can pack on the pounds with carbs and protein, too. According to the National Institute of Health, a "lack of energy balance" is the true culprit behind the obesity crisis. *Energy balance* means that "your energy *in* equals your energy *out*." In other words, don't eat more calories than you burn during the course of the day. From this perspective, fat isn't a villain. Which is a good thing, because, as a runner, you'll need fat in your diet if you want to run well and stay injury-free.

For low- to-moderate-intensity exercise, fat is your body's primary fuel. Its high-density energy makes it a perfect fuel source. The drawback to burning fat is that it takes longer to convert to usable energy than carbohydrates do. That's not a problem when your energy needs are

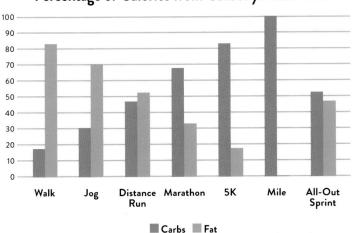

Percentage of Calories from Carbohydrates & Fat

■ Carbs ■ Fat

low, such as when you're sitting down and reading this book. But it can become an issue when your energy needs increase—for example, when you're racing a 5K. When you walk or jog, you rely primarily on fat for energy. But about the time you segue from a normal distance run to a tempo effort, carbohydrates become your primary energy source.

A funny thing happens, however, when you reach an exercise effort equivalent to an all-out sprint or a heavy weight lifting set: Fat becomes your primary energy source again. We first mentioned this phenomenon back in Chapter 6, when we were discussing training for a weight-loss goal. When you exercise at the highest intensity, you use a source of anaerobic energy that's fueled by creatine phosphate and which provides an eight- to fifteen-second burst of high-octane power. Creatine phosphate will provide almost 50 percent of the energy used for a 100-meter dash, and close to 100 percent of the energy burned during a low-rep set of heavy weight lifting. But according to a recent article in the journal *Biology*, authored by exercise scientist Christopher B. Scott, PhD, this depleted creatine phosphate is then reconstituted post-exercise through the breakdown of fat. In fact, during the post-exercise recovery interval, almost *all* of your energy is fueled by fat. This makes high-intensity training a great fat-burning activity.

But including healthy fats in your diet isn't just about energy. Fat also affects both running performance and your chance of getting injured:

RUNNING PERFORMANCE: Two studies, in 2000 and 2001, found that a diet including 30 percent fat led to a 15 to 20 percent improvement in running performance over diets that restricted fat to about 15 percent of total calories. A diet with 40 percent fat provided a similar boost.

INJURY PREVENTION: A 2008 study found that women whose diets included less than 30 percent fat were 250 percent more likely to get injured (e.g., with stress fractures, tendinitis, and iliotibial band syndrome).

If you don't allot 30 percent of your daily calories to fat, you probably won't get the most out of your running program. And if you're training for an event that will take you longer than four hours to complete (e.g., an ultramarathon), you'll want to eat even more fat—as the more fat you eat, the more efficient your body becomes at using it as your primary fuel source.

Protein

Proteins have been called the "building blocks of life." They provide structural and functional support for your cells. They're essential to muscle repair post-workout. And they're the basis of hormones like HGH, which triggers adaptations in your muscles and connective tissue (e.g., bones, tendons, and ligaments), and insulin, which pulls carbohydrates from your bloodstream and deposits them into your muscles. Under normal circumstances, you won't use protein for energy during exercise.

Proteins are made up of amino acids. Your body needs twenty-one different amino acids in order to make *complete proteins*. Your body can make twelve of the amino acids itself; these are called *nonessential* amino acids. There are nine amino acids that you must get from food; these are called *essential* amino acids. Your daily goal is to stockpile all twenty-one amino acids, combining your body's production of nonessential amino acids with the essential ones you get in your food. With this arsenal, your body can create complete proteins, which are then dispatched to support your body's biological functions.

Most animal-based foods provide ready-made complete proteins. These foods include meat, poultry, fish, milk, eggs, and cheese. Most plant-based proteins, like those found in vegetables and grains, are incomplete proteins; to form complete proteins, you'll need to deliver the missing essential amino acids via complementary foods (e.g., rice and beans, cereal and milk, beans and corn, yogurt and granola, tofu and rice, hummus and pita bread, etc.). That said, you don't have to get *all* the essential amino acids in one meal. The prevailing view is that complementary proteins can be consumed throughout the day and still form complete proteins.

If you're an American, you probably already get enough protein in your diet. But just in case, here are the International Society of Sports

Nutrition (ISSN) recommendations for daily protein intake:

ENDURANCE EXERCISE: approximately 0.5 to 0.75 grams of protein per pound of body weight

INTENSE RESISTANCE TRAINING: approximately 0.7 to 0.9 grams of protein per pound of body weight

Since you'll be combining endurance training with some moderate-intensity resistance training, this means you'll need somewhere between 0.5 and 0.9 grams of protein per day per pound of your body weight. As examples, these would be your protein requirements at the following body weights:

→ **100 pounds:** 50 to 90 grams of protein per day

→ **150 pounds:** 75 to 135 grams of protein per day

→ **250 pounds:** 125 to 225 grams of protein per day

You might have heard that diets containing high levels of protein can be dangerous. If you have, you heard wrong. The ISSN has released a position stand on protein and exercise: "Protein intakes [*sic*] of 1.4–2.0 g/kg/day [.6 to .9 grams of protein per pound of body weight per day] is not only safe, but may improve the training adaptations to exercise training."

Bottom line: If you want to improve as a runner, pass the protein.

Vitamins & minerals

If the first thing that popped into your head when you read "vitamins and minerals" was "supplements," think again. When we talk about vitamins and minerals, we're talking about the stuff that comes from *real food*, not from vials of pills on health food store shelves. Real food is food in its original state. It's an apple, not applesauce. It's whole grains, not white bread. It's food pulled straight from the earth, not from a Hostess wrapper. And it has its vitamins and minerals intact. In contrast, processed food often has the nutrition processed right out of it—and is seasoned with extra sugar, extra fat, artificial flavors, and preservatives.

It's a strange world we live in. We buy food that has had the nutrients removed. And then we, as a nation, spend thirty billion dollars per year to get those nutrients back as supplements. On the scary side, supplements aren't regulated (unlike food and over-the-counter medicines), some are spiked with prescription drugs, and they can lead to dangerous vitamin and mineral overdoses.

Better to get your nutrients straight from the source:

VITAMIN B6: important for producing red blood cells and metabolizing protein (*some sources: baked potatoes, bananas, chicken, tuna, salmon, and fortified cereals*)

VITAMIN B12: helps keep your nervous system and red blood cells healthy (*some sources: animal products and fortified vegan products*)

VITAMIN C: an antioxidant that helps protect cells from oxidation (a type of damage), strengthens connective tissue, and boosts the immune system (*some sources: citrus fruits, red and green peppers, broccoli, baked potatoes, and tomatoes*)

VITAMIN D: helps strengthen bones, improves nerve and muscle function, and fortifies your immune system (*some sources: salmon, tuna, eggs, orange juice, and fortified milk and cereals*)

VITAMIN K: high levels lead to better bone density and, possibly, a lower risk of osteoarthritis (*some sources: dark leafy greens, broccoli, brussels sprouts, prunes, avocados, and blueberries*)

CALCIUM: essential for bone strength, but also for muscle contraction, blood pressure regulation, and hormone secretion (*some sources: milk, cheese, yogurt, kale, broccoli, canned sardines, and fortified juices and cereals*)

IRON: essential for red blood cell production and important for growth, immune system function, and metabolism; without adequate amounts, anemia is a risk for runners (*some sources: beef, clams, fortified cereals, oysters, spinach, and kidney beans*)

POTASSIUM: helps regulate nerve and muscle function at the cellular level (*some sources: bananas, baked potatoes, sweet potatoes, milk, cantaloupe, pinto beans, soy products, and peas*)

131,461

SODIUM: helps regulate your body's fluid balance, which affects blood pressure (*some sources: olives, tomato juice, low-fat cottage cheese, and salted nuts*)

When you get your vitamins and minerals from real food, an added bonus is that those foods tend to deliver healthy carbohydrates, fats, and proteins.

GOING ON A DIET

Now that we've discussed the volume of carbohydrates, fats, and proteins you'll need in your running diet (feeling bloated yet?), it's time to turn our attention to the relevant question: How are you going to fit all that nutrition into your diet while simultaneously cutting down calories to shed weight? Hey, if it was easy, between fifty million and one hundred million Americans per year wouldn't be desperately plunking down twenty billion dollars collectively for juice cleanses, stimulants, stomach stapling, liposuction, tube feeding, plastic wrap, colonics, tapeworm treatment, and that old standby, shopping carts full of prepackaged, low-calorie, brand-name diet meals.

First of all, understand that a diet for you, a runner, cannot be *just* about calorie reduction. You could eliminate a lot of calories from your diet by eliminating carbs, but you'd also be sabotaging your running program. Instead, you'll need to pick your calories carefully, ensuring that you maintain a healthy, nutritious diet. And you'll need to implement a long-term weight loss timeline. As with your running goals, your weight loss goal should be to arrive at the finish line eventually, not to cut corners in the hope of arriving day-after-tomorrow.

Determining healthy weight

You'll need to decide how much weight you want to lose—or *if* you need to lose weight at all. While healthy weight loss will lead to better fitness and improved running performance, dieting when you're already thin will simply rob your body of the lean muscle you need to build strength and stay injury-free. A quick way to gauge whether your weight is healthy is to check your Body Mass Index (BMI). Your BMI estimates body fat, and it's calculated from your height and weight. But before checking your

BMI, note that people with muscular builds have higher BMIs without being unhealthy, and older people who've lost lean muscle might have lower BMIs and yet still have higher body fat. To calculate your BMI:

→ Multiply your weight (in pounds) by 703.

→ Divide the answer by your height in inches.

→ Divide again by your height in inches.

If your final answer is between 18.5 and 24.9, then congratulations—you're at a healthy weight! Below 18.5 is underweight. Over 24.9 means you'll need to eliminate the chips and dip from your training diet. If you'd prefer to use an online calculator, just Google "BMI calculator."

If you decide that your BMI is too high (or otherwise conclude that you want to diet), the good news is that there are physical benefits to running at a healthy weight. You'll lower impact forces on your muscles, bones, tendons, and ligaments, resulting in less stiffness and fewer overuse injuries. You'll improve your running economy, leading to better endurance. And you'll enhance your running performance, which means more enjoyable training and better race results.

Of course, regardless of your BMI, only *you* have the final word on your preferred weight. Remember that runners come in all shapes and sizes. The beauty of running isn't reflected by your bathroom mirror; it's experienced on the roads and trails, and it originates from a place beneath the skin—from within your body, mind, and spirit—that no mirror can capture.

Determining healthy weight-loss goals

Rule number one: Be patient.

And, yes, it's hard to be patient when Internet ads, magazines, books, and television personalities are promising that you can "lose 30 pounds in 30 days" or "eat all you want and still lose weight!" But even so, be patient. Fad diets and get-thin-quick schemes won't support your running lifestyle (and won't keep the weight off for long, either). You need energy from carbs and fats to run. You need protein to rebuild your muscles. Nutrients to stay healthy. And you can't get all that on 800 calories a day.

You'll need to think long-term. You'll need to focus on creating a healthier, sustainable lifestyle that *includes* a diet—not one that revolves around your diet. Here are a few guidelines for fashioning your weight loss goal:

→ Shoot for one to two pounds of weight loss per week

→ Aim for a total weight loss of no more than 10 percent of your current weight during the first six months

→ Balance energy in (calories consumed) with energy out (metabolism, exercise, and other physical activity)

→ Maintain a healthy, balanced diet that fully supports your running program

Once you've determined how much weight you want to lose, and once you've decided upon a smart, manageable timeline for your weight loss, it's time to create a diet plan.

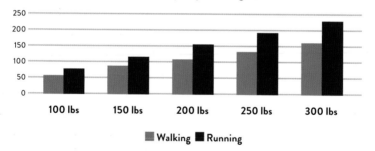

Calories Burned per Mile: Walking & Running
(Based upon your weight)

Beating the spread

The mechanics of losing one to two pounds per week seem simple. There are 3,500 calories in a pound of body fat, so you need to eat 3,500 fewer calories than you expend during a week to lose a pound—7,000 calories to lose two pounds. In other words, you need to run an energy balance deficit of 500 to 1,000 calories per day. Easy, right? Unfortunately, not so easy, as you'll soon see.

You'll begin by calculating the calories you'll need to consume every day to maintain your current weight. This calorie total will be based upon three things:

→ Your body weight

→ Your calorie expenditure during exercise

→ Your basal metabolic rate (the amount of calories expended by your metabolism to keep your body functioning while at rest)

Finding your current weight is a cinch; you can get that from your bathroom scale.

And you can get a rough estimate of the calories you'll burn walking or running by looking at the chart "Calories Burned per Mile: Walking & Running." For a more accurate estimate, use the *Competitor* online calculator, "Calorie Burn Calculator," at: running.competitor.com/pace-calculator.

As for your metabolism, that's a little trickier. Your metabolism accounts for the majority of the calories you'll burn in a day, and it includes the multitude of processes through which your body uses food to create energy and maintain function. But here's where determining your metabolism's contribution to your daily calorie total gets difficult: Your metabolism doesn't have a single setting. Two people with the exact same body weight can have completely different metabolic rates. That's because your metabolism is affected by numerous factors, including your muscle mass, age, gender, hormones, dietary deficiencies, genetics, and body size, as well as by environmental factors like hot and cold weather. There are formulas for determining your resting metabolic rate (e.g., the Mifflin-St Jeor equation, which multiplies your weight in kilograms by your height in centimeters by your age in years, to which you add 5 if you're a man and subtract 161 if you're a woman), but as complicated as those formulas can be, they're still only good guesses. What's more, your metabolism will be significantly affected by three additional factors that are intrinsic to your combination fitness/weight loss program:

1 CALORIE RESTRICTION: Studies consistently show that dieting lowers metabolism. A 1991 study published in the *American Journal of Clinical Nutrition* found that just three weeks of a very low-calorie diet lowered metabolism to 82 percent of normal. And a 2000 study found that lowered metabolism could become at least semipermanent: Eight subjects were confined to a biosphere for two years, during which they lived on a restricted-calorie diet. Six months after leaving the biosphere and returning to a normal diet, the subjects *still* had reduced metabolisms. In other words, as soon as you start feeding your body fewer calories, your body responds by burning fewer calories, and this outcome can continue long after your diet has been abandoned.

2 WEIGHT LOSS: Yes, I know, this doesn't seem fair, but weight loss itself leads to lowered metabolism. This makes sense when you think about it. When there's less of you to maintain, you'll need fewer calories to do it.

3 EXERCISE: This is the good factor, the one that can partially (or wholly) offset the first two. When you exercise, you increase your metabolism *post-exercise*. You do this by creating an *afterburn*—a period of time during which your metabolic calorie usage rises even though you are no longer exercising. While there's debate about how much afterburn you'll experience (higher intensity exercise appears to create a higher afterburn than purely aerobic exercise), there's no doubt that the post-exercise burn will help counter the reduced metabolism that results from calorie restriction and weight loss.

If all of this has your head spinning (i.e., you still have no idea how many calories you should eat, and all this information is just increasing your confusion—maybe you're thinking it's time to grab some comfort pizza and Coca-Cola and delay the diet indefinitely), I'd counsel you to relax. You won't need a pencil and paper to figure this out. Instead, you can use an online calculator to estimate your daily caloric needs, based upon body weight, height, age, and sex. Some online calculators:

→ **My Fitness Pal:** myfitnesspal.com/tools/bmr-calculator

→ **Bodybuilding.com:** bodybuilding.com/fun/bmr_calculator.htm

Next, add the calories you'll expend exercising. Both of these calculators should give you a close estimate of your exercise-induced calorie burn:

→ **Competitor Calorie Burn Calculator:** running.competitor. com/pace-calculator

→ **My Fitness Pal Calories Burned from Exercise:** myfitnesspal.com/exercise/lookup

Once you know how many calories you require to maintain your current weight, you'll need to adjust that total downward in order to lose weight. A reduction of 500 to 1,000 calories per day should result in a healthy weight loss of one to two pounds per week. If you don't see weight loss by the third or fourth week, you'll need to adjust your caloric intake downward a little more until you do.

If you prefer to have an online calculator do *all* the diet planning for you, try the "Body Weight Planner," provided by the National Institutes of Health. The BWP first calculates your metabolic rate and daily activity, and then it determines the calories necessary for maintaining your current weight *and* the calorie reduction required to reach your goal weight. Better still, you can input the exact date you want to reach your target weight, and the BWP will adjust your daily calorie total to help you reach that goal. The one drawback to the BWP is that is doesn't calculate exact caloric expenditure for your exercise; it simply slots you into a generic category based upon overall physical activity. To try out the BWP:

→ **NIH Body Weight Planner:** supertracker.usda.gov/bwp/index. html

Finally, do *not* panic if you don't see weight loss in the first one or two weeks. Your body increases your muscle glycogen stores when you first start training, adding one to four pounds of good carbohydrate (and accompanying water) weight—a gain that might offset early weight loss from your diet.

Making your calories count

Once you know your daily calorie allotment, you'll want to put together a nutritional plan that doesn't sabotage your running. In doing so, you'll need to merge two diet goals:

RUNNING DIET GOAL: Eat enough carbs, fats, proteins, vitamins, and minerals to ensure that you'll have the energy and nutrition to train, recover, and adapt

WEIGHT LOSS GOAL: Lower your calorie intake by 500–1,000 calories per day

It's the skillful synthesis of these competing goals that will determine the success of both your diet and running program.

The obvious first step is to eliminate highly processed, nutrient-deficient foods from your diet. You'll replace these with real food: vegetables, dark leafy greens, bright fruits, beans, whole grains, nuts, avocados, cheese, yogurt, fish, poultry, lean meat, eggs, etc. Stay away from white flour and white sugar. Embrace wheat pasta and brown rice. You can ensure variety in your diet by eating seasonal foods (e.g., for fruit, strawberries in the spring, peaches and cherries in the summer, and apples and pears in the fall). With real food, you'll get better nutrition from fewer calories.

Next, add up your carbs, fats, and proteins. Make sure you're getting enough of each. If you're getting *more than enough* of any one of them, that's a good place to cut some calories.

Finally, don't forget your post-workout snack of carbohydrates and protein. Not only will that have your legs feeling fresh for the next workout, it will stave off post-workout hunger.

Planning your pre-run fueling

Another decision you'll have to make concerns pre-run fueling. We briefly touched on this topic in Chapter 10, noting that most runners train best on an empty stomach. When you run, not only is blood shunted away from your stomach and intestines toward your working muscles, but the very act of running jostles food in your digestive tract, speeding it along its way. For many runners who've eaten too much or too soon before their workout, the result is runner's trots (i.e., cramping and a pressing need to defecate, often multiple times). Trust me, you don't want to experience this. Personally, I don't eat or drink for about three hours before training or racing. But I've coached runners who are perfectly happy eating a small meal within minutes of setting off on a run. Most runners do best somewhere in the middle: They eat an easily digestible snack a couple hours before their run, while consuming just enough water to maintain hydration (avoiding overhydration). You'll need to experiment to discover what works best for you. But remember: A race is *never* the time to experiment; fueling strategies should always be tested prior to normal training runs.

Plumping while running

It would be remiss of me to leave this chapter without mentioning one other argument that regularly arises regarding the combination of diet and exercise: namely, that exercise programs lead to weight *gain*, not weight loss. These arguments, often promoted by the media or non-exercise-based diet programs, cite studies that have found weight gain among walkers, joggers, or other dieters in exercise programs. The thing to understand is that *none* of these studies reflects the specific effect of exercise itself upon weight gain; instead, they reflect the fact that people who exercise get hungry—and then some of these same people overeat. In fact, studies have found that people who exercise often overestimate the amount of calories they're burning (during exercise) by two to three times. It's no wonder that when these same people subsequently eat twice (or thrice) the calories required to offset that burn, they gain weight. You wouldn't expect to run three miles, burn 300 calories, and then lose weight by chasing your run with a Baskin Robbins 800-calorie Warm Brownie Sundae. This is all the more reason to work out an accurate daily calorie total—and then to make incremental adjustments until you meet your weight-loss goal.

As runners, we sometimes treat our bodies as if they were our enemy. As if their inability to transform at faster than an incremental rate is a betrayal, is a direct challenge to our authority and aspirations. But our bodies aren't the enemy. Our bodies quite literally *are* us—or, at least, our physical incarnation on this planet, for this life. And treating our bodies with respect—with the recognition that they are flesh and blood, and fragile, and capable of only gradual, step-by-step change—is akin to treating ourselves with the same respect. It took you a lifetime to become

BECOMING A RUNNER: *Marisa Pearson*

Marisa Pearson, age forty-three, of North Hollywood, California, started running in 2013 when Tony's Darts Away, one of her favorite pubs, offered a two-dollar beer discount to finishers of a local 5K. She and some friends ran the race. Drank some beer. And agreed they'd run really badly. So they signed up for a Fleet Feet 5K training program. Marisa, a casting director for commercials, didn't exactly have a fitness background—no high school or college sports, and no gym work except for a few years of once-a-week Pilates. But she enjoyed running, and the 5K program soon segued to a 10K program, and then to marathon training with Coach Larry. "But I just kept getting injury after injury," says Marisa. In January of 2014, during a Spartan Sprint race, Marisa hurt her knee doing burpees on the sand hills. Her doctor ordered an X-ray of her knee and hip. "That's when they found the stress line in my hip," she says. Next, she got a bone-density scan. "By 6:45 that same night," says Marisa, "I got the call saying I had osteoporosis." In fact, she had idiopathic osteoporosis, a relatively rare disorder in which otherwise young, healthy individuals develop weak and brittle bones. Scared to death, with a half marathon scheduled for that weekend and having just signed up for her first marathon, Marisa saw both a rheumatologist and an endocrinologist. The news wasn't what she wanted to hear: *Consider walking the half marathon—because no one knows how strong your bones are.* Marisa rejected the advice. "I was thinking who you are, and it will take time now to become the person you want to be. Whether that's running a 5K or losing a few pounds, the best path is the one that actually takes you to your destination. Shortcuts are rarely shortcuts; more often, they're beelines back to the start line. Be patient with weight loss. Your body isn't a toy with which to trifle. It's you. And you're worth the effort, no matter how long it takes.

that I might not have twenty years of running like most people my age," she says, explaining her rationale. Besides, she'd run a half dozen half marathons the previous year, probably a few with the cracked hip. So she went ahead and ran the half marathon. It went fine. And then, on her forty-third birthday, in November 2014, Marisa ran her first marathon. It, too, was a success. A few half marathons later, she still hasn't stress-fractured. And she has already registered for next year's Big Sur Marathon. Not that she hasn't adjusted her training. "I don't care about speed anymore," she says. "I don't care if I PR in races anymore." Still, the news isn't all good. A recent bone-density scan showed little improvement in her condition, if any. And an MRI to check Marisa's pituitary gland (to rule out its involvement with her osteoporosis) revealed a healthy pituitary but picked up "white spots" throughout her brain—a mystery for which there is not yet a solution. But Marisa isn't giving up. And she intends to keep doing what she wants to do, sports-wise, for as long as she can do it. "I was brought up, something's only a handicap if you let it be one," she says. "You can't let other peoples' fears rule your behavior. You have to live your life."

CHAPTER TAKEAWAY

The primary feature of your running diet must be this: You must get enough of the nutrition you require—the carbs, fats, proteins, vitamins, and minerals—to successfully perform your running program. Understanding how each macronutrient and nutrient contributes to your overall fitness will help you to determine the amount of each to include in your daily diet. If you also have a goal of healthy weight loss (i.e., dieting), you'll have to determine the total daily calories your body needs (by considering your body weight, metabolism, and daily exercise) and then reduce those calories by the amount required to shed one to two pounds per week. In doing so, you'll have to balance your running program energy and nutritional needs with your weight-loss goal. As with your running program goals, you'll need to think long-term and practice patience.

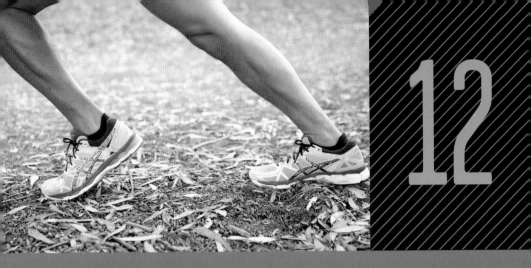

12

Injury Prevention 101

"Even monkeys fall from trees."
—JAPANESE SAYING

BETWEEN THE AGES OF FORTY-TWO AND FORTY-FOUR, I slept with a crutch at my bedside. I was suffering from plantar fasciitis, an injury that's been compared to having a nail hammered into your heel with every step (sounds about right to me), and an injury that is most painful after a night's sleep. Without the crutch, I would have had to crawl on all fours in the morning. As it was, I'd hang on to the crutch through breakfast, keep it while I showered and dressed, and then finally leave it by the front door as I exited for work. By then, I'd warmed up enough to limp through the day. And by late afternoon, I was ready to grit my teeth through a distance run, repetitions, or whatever was on the schedule. I did that for three years. And then one day the pain was just too much, forcing me to quit in the middle of my workout. I took five months off, and the pain went away. So I laced up my shoes, headed out the door, and made it almost a mile before pain shot through my heel, jolting me so badly that I tasted iron on my tongue. My plantar fascia hadn't healed. Time off hadn't worked. If I was going to run again, I'd need a different plan. So this is what I did: I designed a routine to strengthen the tendons, muscles, and ligaments around my plantar fascia, to ease the stress on the injured tissue. Every day, I did towel toe curls, foot orbits, rope stretching, and more. Within a week, I could run with reduced pain. Within a month, I could train again. And three months later, I won the 2005 USA masters 10K cross country championship.

Injury prevention isn't just the art of avoiding injuries. It's also a plan of action: You strengthen your body to reduce the possibility of injury and to minimize the effects when injuries occur. And injuries do occur. Between 50 and 80 percent of runners get injured every year. But before you get alarmed, probably 90 to 99 percent of those injured runners don't include injury-prevention exercises (or any kind of resistance training) in their programs. Maybe they don't think they're training hard enough to bother with injury prevention. Maybe they don't think they have enough time. Whatever the excuse, it's almost a given that runners who ignore the possibility of injury *will* get injured.

Luckily, most non-acute injuries develop slowly, and there are usually warning signs. For plantar fasciitis, it's a sharp pain in your heel. For Achilles tendinitis, it might be tight calves. Iliotibial (IT) band syndrome can be preceded by a prickly feeling on the outside of your knee. For these types of injuries—and for chronic injuries that need to be resolved—the injury-prevention exercises after this chapter can offer immunization and relief.

This chapter will help you to understand running injuries, identify them, prevent them, and, if necessary, rehabilitate them. For smart runners, what follows isn't just Injury Prevention 101; it's Basic Training 101.

ARE YOU REALLY INJURED?

Not every ache is an injury. Most runners can expect to feel some aches and pains during their first weeks of training. That's because your transformation from nonathlete to runner requires a full-body rebuild. You damage muscles, bones, and tendons in order to repair them so that they're stronger than they were before. That's going to engender the occasional owie.

So when should you worry?

That's a good question. And to answer it, we'll examine a few types of injuries, and we'll suggest some guidelines for dealing with different injury scenarios.

STOP RUNNING IMMEDIATELY!

While infrequent, there are emergency situations that arise while running. Emergency situations include life-threatening health conditions, serious accidents (e.g., collisions with cars), and severe and debilitating injuries (e.g., a badly sprained ankle or muscle tear). In these instances, you should immediately end your workout. And then don't be shy. If the situation warrants, find someone nearby—even if it means flagging down a car or knocking on a door (unless your physical condition precludes walking)—and get the help you need. When these emergency situations occur, you should:

→ Call 911 if you suffer chest pain that persists for more than a minute, spreads to your neck or shoulders, or is accompanied by severe sweating or faintness. Stop immediately and alert someone nearby. It might not be a heart attack, but better safe than sorry.

→ Seek immediate medical attention if you suffer heart arrhythmia, breathing difficulties, disorientation, sudden cessation of sweating (heat stroke), severe fever or headache, badly blurred vision, or other potentially life-threatening symptoms. Also, if you're struck by a car or suffer some other major accident, you'll need to be checked out pronto by a health professional—if the situation warrants, refer to the advice directly above: *Call 911.*

→ See your doctor if you suffer a stress fracture, meniscus tear, torn tendon or ligament, or some other structural damage. Do *not* walk home if you're on a run. Wait for a ride.

→ Consider seeing a health professional if you suffer a sudden or severe muscle injury (sharp or debilitating pain) while training. Do *not* walk home if you're on a run. Wait for a ride.

Common types of injuries

Next, let's break down the types of running injuries that occur. Most runners will deal with each of the following four classifications of injuries. When reading through them, see if you can spot the common thread. (Answer: They all begin with runner error).

OVERUSE INJURIES: You do the same exercise over and over (e.g., all same-pace distance running), which leads to irritation of some tissue (e.g., runner's knee).

OVERLOAD INJURIES: You increase the volume or intensity of your exercise too quickly, triggering acute inflammation (e.g., DOMS, Achilles tendinitis, etc.).

CHRONIC INJURIES: These develop when you ignore minor overuse or overload injuries, creating degenerative damage in the affected area that simply won't go away (e.g., Achilles tendinosis).

ACCIDENTS: Single incidents that stop your workout in its tracks. You step on a rock and sprain your ankle. Or jam your toe, pull a hamstring, trip and fracture your wrist, and so on. The best way to avoid accidents is to pay attention—always remain 100 percent aware of your surroundings, foot placement, and fatigue levels (tired runners tend to trip, kick things, and step in potholes).

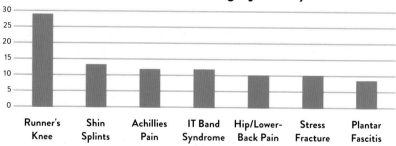

Most Common Running Injuries (by %)

No one wants to curtail his or her training due to injury. But the sooner you address the situation, the sooner you can put it behind you. Many long-term injuries begin as minor ones and can be remedied by preventative care. You've heard the old saying, *A stitch in time saves nine*. Well, in this case, the "stitch" is your injury-prevention exercises, and the "nine" represents the days, weeks, or months you'll spend on the couch if you ignore the warning signs.

Assessing common injuries and syndromes

Of course, once you've accepted that something is wrong, the next step is to decide whether it's *really* wrong (in which case you should end your workout) or just sort of wrong (you can continue your workout). The ability to correctly assess the severity of your injury will help keep your training program on track. By recognizing that an injury is minor, you'll be able to continue training and won't sacrifice fitness. At the same time, you won't ignore major injuries, a mistake that can land you back on the couch for an extended stay.

SUDDEN PAIN: If you experience sudden pain while running, you'll want to do two things. First, stop exercising—*immediately*. Second, if the pain subsides, walk for a minute or two to ensure that you haven't broken, twisted, sprained, strained, or otherwise damaged the area that's hurting. If you can walk comfortably, try jogging; if jogging is OK, then gradually return to your previous pace. If you can't walk without pain—and if the pain just won't go away—then it's time to end your workout. Find a phone, call a friend, family member, or cab, and wait for a ride home.

MUSCLE SORENESS: If your muscles are so sore that it's torture to exercise, you'll need to take the day off. If you recently performed an extremely hard workout, or if you're a new runner who overdid your first workout(s), you probably have DOMS (see page 236 for advice on treating DOMS). If your soreness came on suddenly, you might have a strained muscle; this generally requires time off until the muscle heals.

MUSCLE CRAMPS: If you experience a cramp (most often in your calves or hamstrings) during a run, you'll need to stop running until the cramp subsides. Running with a cramp can result in more serious muscle strains (see page 254 for advice on treating muscle cramps). If you suffer heat-related cramps, you'll need to end your workout (see page 243 for advice on heat illness).

INFLAMMATION: If you notice inflammation that's *not* related to a recent injury, such as swelling in your feet or lower legs (often experienced by people who work at desks), use your fingers to press and probe the affected area. If there's soreness or pain (or if the inflammation is severe), take the day off. If there's no pain and only mild swelling, you can attempt your workout—start with walking, then jogging, then easy running, and quit if you develop pain. If the inflammation persists or worsens, consider seeing a health professional.

LONG-TERM PAIN: If you've been running through a painful condition that's persisted for days, weeks, or even months—and if the condition has *not* gotten worse during that time—you can continue to train as long as you add injury-prevention exercises to your routine. If the symptoms don't get better within a month or two, you'll need to consult a health professional or take time off. You don't want to develop a chronic injury, which can last for years—or *forever.*

ALTERING YOUR STRIDE DUE TO PAIN: This one is easy: Don't do it. If pain forces you to alter your stride, you need to stop running. Your stride represents movement that is biomechanically correct for your body. Changing your stride creates movement that is biomechanically incorrect. The result will be yet another injury.

LIGHTHEADEDNESS: Sometimes, we runners get lightheaded. This can be caused by low blood sugar, low muscle glycogen (carbohydrates stored in your muscles), dehydration, extreme fatigue, post-caffeine crash (for those who like a cup of Joe pre-run), or various types of anxiety. If you suspect low blood sugar or low muscle glycogen, pop a gel (or some other carbohydrate snack). If dehydration, drink some water. Whatever the cause, you'll want to walk until the dizziness goes away. Then restart your run at a reduced effort level. If the dizziness persists, you might consider seeing a health professional to rule out anemia, diabetes, or some other condition.

For advice specific to individual injuries, see the "Identify Your Running Injury" table in this chapter (page 223) and proceed to the pages indicated for further information and injury-prevention instruction.

WHAT NOT TO DO

It's also important to know what *not* to do when pain, inflammation, or other symptoms of injury strike. First, never panic. You might not even be injured. If you were to slap your hand on your thigh, both your hand and your thigh would sting for a few seconds; that doesn't mean either is injured. Same goes for momentary stinging, tingling, throbbing, and other discomfort on the roads and trails—after all, each stride creates an impact force that's two to three times your body weight, adding up to one hundred to three hundred tons of impact force (depending on your weight) per mile. The occasional niggle or twinge is to be expected. Second, if you think that you really *are* injured, resist the following debunked strategies for dealing with your injury:

STRETCHING: Your parents always told you not to pick at scabs. Don't stretch a freshly injured muscle (muscle cramps excluded), tendon, or ligament, either—not without guidance from a physical therapist or other health professional.

ICING: Icing relieves pain, but it also interrupts the body's normal healing process. For minor muscle injuries and inflammation, don't do it. For more serious injuries or inflammation that's spiraling out of control, ice for the first 24–48 hours (12–15 minutes at a time).

HEAT: Never in the first 24 hours following an acute injury, as you'll only increase inflammation. Wait two or three days before turning to heat therapy.

ANTI-INFLAMMATORIES: Like icing, anti-inflammatories can theoretically interrupt the normal healing process for muscles. That said, studies have shown increased strength gains in older runners who use ibuprofen (e.g., Advil) or the pain-reliever acetaminophen (e.g., Tylenol). A cautious approach for all runners would be to limit the use of anti-inflammatories to instances of significant pain or immobility.

ANTIOXIDANT SUPPLEMENTS: Yes, antioxidants (e.g., vitamin C, selenium, and flavonoids) can reduce the damage that free radicals (pesky atoms and molecules that can form during exercise) inflict on your cells. But that doesn't mean that antioxidant supplements are helpful. Recent studies have linked antioxidant supplementation to accelerated lung, prostate, and skin (melanoma) cancer and have debunked anecdotal claims for cardiovascular health benefits. Of specific concern for runners, these supplements can partially negate the minor damage required to stimulate improvement in your muscles.

"SHAKE IT OFF": You can't "shake off" a pulled hamstring or a stress fracture. Don't listen to anyone who advises differently.

Before you decide that running is simply *too scary* a sport to endure, what with the multitude of injuries lurking around every corner, understand that most injuries aren't serious. They're bumps in the road. Yes, you might have to deal with a sore spot here and there. But, overall, your training will leave you feeling *much* healthier and more energetic. And, as explained previously, you'll increase your odds (dramatically!) of avoiding major hip, knee, and disability issues that affect non-runners. Plus, the injury-prevention exercises after this chapter can help immunize you against many common injuries. Consider them a form of prescient healing—as reinforcement for your body's various Achilles' heels before injury can strike.

INCORPORATING INJURY-PREVENTION EXERCISES INTO YOUR PROGRAM

If you do decide to schedule injury-prevention exercises, you'll need to know when and how often to perform the exercises. The easiest plan is to add the injury-prevention exercises to your strength training program (e.g., the Beginner's Body Strengthening routine on page 275). If you do your strength program twice a week, that should be enough. If you only include a strength program once per week (or don't schedule one at all), you'll still want to perform your injury-prevention exercises at least twice a week (three times is better). The best time for scheduling injury-prevention exercises is directly after easy distance runs, when your muscles are warmed up. You don't want to perform your exercises after a high-intensity workout, as your muscles and connective tissue will already be fatigued.

FINAL THOUGHTS—AND THEN OUT THE DOOR WITH YOU

We've all seen werewolf movies, watched a bitten human endure the curse of bones elongating and skin stretching and organs becoming engorged with new mass, the afflicted person screaming in agony during the hideous transmogrification.

The good news is that you're not becoming a werewolf. You're becoming a runner. And while your transformation will be equally all-encompassing, it will be gradual. Any discomfort you experience will be short-lived and manageable. And the only scream to emerge from your throat will be one of triumph as you achieve your personal running goal.

And now, before I leave you to the injury-prevention photo instruction in this chapter—and then to the Beginner's Body Strenthening routing and the acknowledgments and the index—I'd like to share one last thing about running.

What I'd like to share is this: The best part of becoming a runner is *not* the physical transformation you'll experience. And it's not achieving your running goals. If goals were all there was to running, millions of people wouldn't have made the sport a lifestyle. They would have made it a fad, like ThighMaster, stripper aerobics, the Shake Weight, and Tae Bo. But they didn't. And that's because, at its core, running isn't a sport of fleeting fitness gains; it's a sport of universal and transcendent intangibles. It's the courage to start a program. And the patience and perseverance to stick with it. It's the passion we bring to chasing our goals. And our pride when we achieve them. It's inspiration and discipline, and exhilaration and disappointment. And sometimes it's pain. And other times it's joy.

But mostly, for me, it's gratitude—gratitude that the simple act of running allowed me to reclaim my health, my fitness, and, most importantly, my relationship with my son. Gratitude that in my fifties, I can function fully as a physical being. Gratitude for the nomadic freedom of my daily runs. And gratitude for the ineffable spirit that running has laid bare, the vital blend of body and mind that I experience every day, and for the interconnectedness I've discovered between that spirit and the world through which I travel.

BECOMING A RUNNER: *Eric Dixon*

Eric Dixon, of Buena Park, California, who at age fifty-six is one of the world's top age-group sprinters, didn't run in high school. "I always wanted to," he says. "But I couldn't run for a track team because everyone would see the bruises on my body." For Eric, the beatings from his mother and father began when he was two years old and continued through his teenage years. Once, he was locked in a basement closet for four days without food. Another time, his mother hog-tied and beat him all day. Three times, he attempted suicide, twice with pills and once by walking with his eyes closed into a busy street. The abuse finally ended on New Year's Day, 1978, when his father shot his mother dead in front of Eric. After briefly turning to gangs and drugs, Eric joined the Air Force. He was stationed in Germany, and, finally ready to run, challenged the Air Force's top sprinter at Ramstein Air Base to a race. "I kicked his butt," says Eric. And so he found himself on the Air Force track team. At a meet in Frankfurt, Eric posted a time of 10.05 for 100 meters, ranking him as one of the top sprinters in the world. A scholarship offer from the University of Maryland brought him back to the States, but it wasn't to be. Crossing the street, on his way to a summer job in Washington, DC, Eric was struck by a car traveling sixty miles per hour. His lower left leg was shattered. "It looked like Cap'n Crunch's Crunch Berry cereal," says Eric. His doctor gave Eric a 5 to 10 percent chance of walking again—and no chance to run. "I told him I was going

I believe that you, too, will come to understand that your running body is not merely a body, that the souped-up, flesh-and-blood machine you'll create is instead an incarnation of something bigger—of the change you'll bring into your life, the optimism that will fuel your days, and the gift that will define your path forward: *control of your own destiny.*

to run," says Eric. And he meant it. He'd felt helpless during the years of child abuse. Through running, Eric had regained control of his life. "I wasn't giving up," he says. With ten rods in his leg, secured by a Hoffman External Fixator, Eric started rehab, doing leg curls and leg extensions. More than a year later, the Hoffman was replaced with a long cast, and six months after that with a short cast. "I would do a lot of meditating," says Eric, "visualizing my leg healing." After two years, he could walk. A year after that, he was able to increase the intensity of his training. But it would be decades before he regained top form as a masters runner, claiming world age-group top-ten performances in the 100m, 200m, and 400m races. Along the way, he'd claim even greater non-running achievements, rearing his son Ryan, now twenty-one, in a loving household, and working with the Wounded Warrior Project, using his experience to help injured veterans find physical and psychological healing. Eric's message for all injured warriors, veteran and civilian, is the same: "If I can come back from this, then you can come back from yours."

CHAPTER TAKEAWAY

Injuries happen. Between 50 and 80 percent of runners experience them each year. But as shocking as that number might seem, it doesn't tell the whole story. Because injuries are *not* inevitable. A good all-around resistance training routine, smart running, and injury-prevention exercises to preempt potential injuries can keep your running program on track. Also, not all aches and pains are injuries. Sometimes, they're just aches and pains. Success in a long-term running program requires the ability to discern between transient discomfort and actual injury—and then the willingness to address injury with action, with exercises to strengthen the injured tissue and all supporting muscles, tendons, and ligaments.

Identify Your Running Injury

FEET & ANKLES	Achilles Pain	224	Pain experienced behind your heel or along the tendon running from your heel to the base of your calf
	Ankle Sprain	228	Pain, inflammation, discoloration, and reduced mobility of the ankle
	Black Toenails	232	Painful, discolored (black/purple) toenails
	Blisters	232	A sometimes-painful bubble of fluid trapped beneath the skin
	Bunions	233	A bony bump at the base of your big toe that can be red and sore
	Plantar Fasciitis	258	Pain that can be felt at the point where the heel meets the arch but that is often first felt as pain on the bottom of the heel
	Stress Fracture (Metatarsal)	274	Sharp pain in your foot that can be felt over a wide area but is sharper and more intense when pressure is applied directly to the spot of the fracture
LOWER LEGS	Calf Strain	233	Pain and tightness in your calves
	Shin Splints (Front)	266	Sharp pain along the outside (front) of your shin(s)
	Shin Splints (Medial)	268	Sharp pain along the inside (medial location) of your shin(s)
	Stress Fracture (Tibia)	274	Sharp pain along your shin (feels like severe shin splints) that hurts from the first step of your run until the last
KNEES	IT Band Syndrome	246	Pain on either the outside of your knee (usually) or the outside of your hip (less frequently) generated by a tight IT band or by weak hip and glute muscles
	Knee Pain (General)	249	Generalized, sharp knee pain that can occur on the front of the knee without an obvious inciting incident or visible swelling or damage
	Meniscus Tear	253	Pain at the side or center of the knee, accompanied by swelling and usually following a twisting motion
	Osteoarthritis	256	Pain, swelling, and immobility in a joint (for runners, usually knee or hip) caused by a loss of cartilage
	Runner's Knee	262	Knee pain emanating from beneath your kneecap
HIP, THIGHS & GROIN	Chafing	236	Painful irritation of the skin caused by rubbing against skin or fabric
	DOMS	236	Muscular pain following changes in training intensity or duration
	Groin Strain	237	Pain in the groin or inner-thigh area, especially when lifting your knee
	Hamstring Strain	240	Pain or tightness in your hamstring (back of thigh), often restricting movement
	Heavy Legs	244	A sense of heaviness and unresponsiveness in the legs; low energy
	Hip Pain	244	Nonspecific pain in the hip area
	Muscle Cramps/ Hamstrings & Calves	254	Sudden, involuntary, and sustained contraction of a muscle that causes pain and doesn't relax
	Piriformis Syndrome	256	Sharp pain, tingling, or numbness that originates slightly above the center-middle portion of your glutes (buttocks)
	Quadriceps Pain	261	Aching, painful quadriceps (front thigh) muscles that isn't related to DOMS or some other inciting incident
	Sciatica	263	Pain, tingling (pins and needles) and/or numbness that is usually felt in the lower back, buttocks, and hamstrings, but can radiate down through the calves and feet
ABOVE THE WAIST	Heat Illness	243	Overheating due to high temperatures, high humidity, or hard training; induces cramps, nausea, headache, weakness. Heat stroke, the most severe heat illness, is a life-threatening condition with high fever, red skin, confusion, rapid pulse, seizures, and unconsciousness.
	Lower-Back Pain & Stiffness	252	Pain or stiffness in the lower back
	Side Stitch	270	A sharp pain just beneath the rib cage (usually on the right side, but can occur on the left side as well)

INJURY-PREVENTION EXERCISES:
PHOTO INSTRUCTION

IF YOU DETERMINE that specific injury-prevention exercises should be part of your program, you'll want to schedule them two to three times per week. They can be added to your regular strength training routine or performed separately, with the optimum time being the first fifteen to thirty minutes after easy distance runs (while your muscles are still warm and supple from the run).

For an illustrated and interactive guide to help diagnose your injury, you can visit my website—petemagill.com—and click the link for the "Interactive Runner," or you can access the Interactive Runner directly at: petemagill.com/interactive-runner/#/irunner. The resistance bands, resistance tubing, and wobble board featured in some of the following exercises are available from Thera-Band, sporting goods stores, or online vendors (just Google them).

ACHILLES PAIN

Achilles pain is experienced in several ways. Achilles bursitis is an inflammation of the bursa that acts as cushioning between the Achilles tendon and where the tendon inserts at the heel. Achilles tendinitis is an overuse injury accompanied by painful inflammation in the Achilles tendon. And Achilles tendinosis involves degenerative damage in the Achilles tendon that produces chronic pain without inflammation (this is the cause of most Achilles pain). The decision to run while experiencing Achilles pain should be based on the type and intensity of the pain: Runners who experience Achilles tendinitis will need to take a few days off, while those with tendinosis or bursitis might choose to train (unless the pain becomes incapacitating). The following exercises can help prevent all three conditions (and are great for rehabbing Achilles bursitis and Achilles tendinosis).

Heel dips

Heel dips affect your Achilles tendon directly, strengthening this connective tissue.

1 Use the balls of your feet to balance on a platform with your heels extending over the edge. Then put all of your weight on one foot and slowly lower the heel of that foot toward the floor (through your full range of motion). Beginners or runners with significant flexibility issues with their Achilles tendons can start on a flat surface (e.g., the floor), rising up on their toes and then lowering the heel until it reaches the flat surface; after a few weeks, they can switch to using a platform. You should always use a chair or other support for balance.

2 Use both feet to rise back up, then repeat. As you become stronger, hold a weight (e.g., a dumbbell) in the same-side hand as the heel you're lowering. Increase the weight as your strength increases. Start with 2–5 repetitions for each foot. Gradually build up to 3 sets of 20 repetitions for each foot and perform the exercise 3–5 times per week.

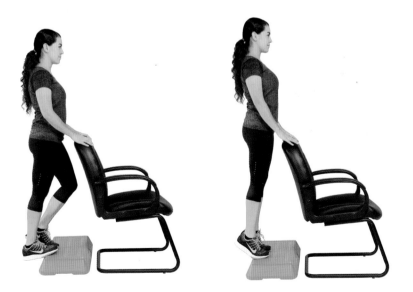

AIS calves

This stretching exercise increases the range of motion for your gastroc-nemius muscle (the largest muscle in your calf), relieving stress on your Achilles tendon.

1 Sit with one leg extended in front of you, the other bent. Loop your rope around the ball of your foot.

2 Use the muscles of your lower leg—specifically, the muscle on the outside (front) of your shin—to pull the ball of your foot toward your shin (bending at the ankle). When you can't pull your foot any closer to your shin, use the rope to gently pull your foot just a tiny bit more (never beyond your natural range of motion). Don't hold the stretch for more than a single second; then immediately return to your starting position. Do 10 reps, then switch sides.

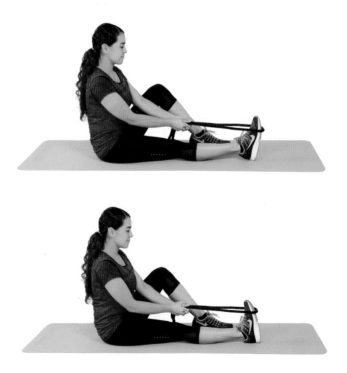

Heel lift

For Achilles tendinitis, some runners get relief by placing a heel lift into their shoe (use athletic tape on the bottom of the lift to hold it in place). The lift should be ⅛ to ¼ inch cork or felt. Don't use for more than a few days, and remove the heel lift as soon as the pain goes away.

Remove shoe heel counter

For Achilles bursitis (pain on the very back of the heel that can radiate to the ankle and bottom of the heel), you might consider performing surgery on your running shoe. Many shoes have extremely rigid heel counters (the plastic insert reinforcing the heel cup of your shoe); these heel counters can aggravate the Achilles tendon at its insertion point. Cutting off the upper back portion of this counter or carving out a big piece of it over the inflamed heel area can go a long way to reducing the pain of this injury. You'll need a box cutter or other sharp instrument to perform this shoe surgery.

ANKLE SPRAIN

An ankle sprain involves pain, inflammation, discoloration, and reduced mobility of the ankle due to torn (or partially torn) ligaments. For severe ankle sprains, you'll need to see a health professional. To help prevent ankle sprains (if you've sprained your ankle previously, you're more likely to do it again) and to strengthen your ankle after the sprain has healed, try the following exercises.

Balance on one foot

This is the simplest balance exercise of all. Beginners can wear shoes. Once you can balance on one foot for 30 seconds, try it with bare feet.

Stand straight with your knees slightly bent. Lift one foot off the floor and hold it. When you can't balance any longer, put your foot down. Do a single rep of up to 60 seconds on both sides.

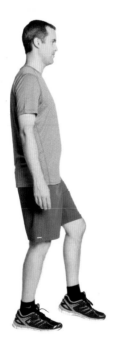

Foot work

These easy-to-do exercises improve your nervous system's control of the muscles responsible for movement at your ankles.

1 Lie on your back with one leg straight, toes pointed upward, and one leg raised and bent 90° at the knee. Prop up the raised leg with your hands.

2 Make circular orbits with your foot, doing 10 rotations clockwise and then 10 rotations counterclockwise. Limit movement to your ankle and foot. After performing the rotations, move your foot backward and forward—toward your shin and then away from it—as if working the gas pedal in your car. Again, do 10 reps with each foot.

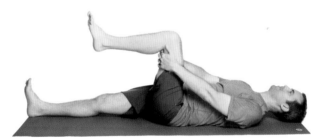

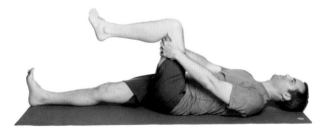

Wobble board

Wobble board training has been shown to reduce the recurrence of ankle sprains by almost 50 percent. It also helps to immunize your body against most knee, lower leg, and foot injuries.

1 Hold on to a chair or other support for balance. Center your weight over the middle of the wobble board. Then rock forward to touch the front of the wobble board to the floor—or as close as you can get. Limit the bend at your knee and focus on working your ankle's range of motion.

2 Rock backward until you touch the floor—or as close as you can get. One rep includes both the forward and backward rock. Begin with 5–10 reps, then increase your reps over time to a maximum of 50.

3 After forward/backward rocking, rock side to side. First, rock inward and touch the side of the wobble board to the floor—or as close as you can get.

4 Next rock outward until you touch the floor—or as close as you can get. One rep includes both the inward and outward rock. Begin with 5–10 reps, then increase your reps over time to a maximum of 50.

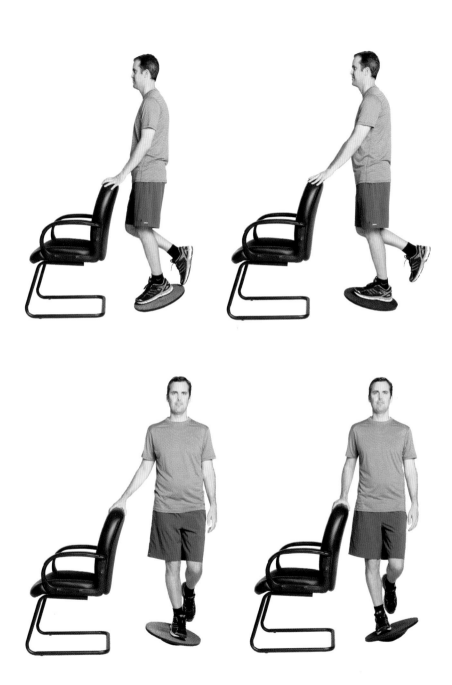

BLACK TOENAILS

Black toenails are painful, discolored (e.g., black or purple) toenails. The toenail is lifted from its bed by fluid or blood buildup. Eventually, it will probably fall off on its own, at which point you can apply antibiotic ointment and a Band-Aid. If the toe becomes red and painful, it might be infected, at which point you should see a health professional. As long as the pain isn't too intense, you can run with black toenails (pretty much every elite runner in the world does—personally, half my toenails are usually black or missing).

BLISTERS

A blister is a (sometimes painful) bubble of fluid trapped beneath the skin that is caused by friction and irritation. For runners, blisters on the feet are a concern. Running on a blister can lead to tearing the blister open—not a pleasant training experience, and one that can lead to infection. By using the following two techniques, you should be able to continue running while the blister heals.

Moleskin, sterilized gauze, athletic tape

You can build up the area surrounding the blister so that you don't put pressure directly on the affected area during a run.

Cut small pieces of moleskin (or other sticky padding) and apply on both sides of a blister (must stack higher than the blister). Wrap sterilized gauze around your foot and across the top of the moleskin/blister. Wrap athletic tape on top of the gauze to hold it in place.

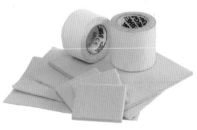

Needle & antibiotic ointment

If you're not squeamish, reducing the size of the blister can negate the problem.

Use a sterilized needle or pin to puncture the blister at its outside edge. Push gently on the blister to drain it. Then apply antibiotic ointment and, if necessary, a bandage.

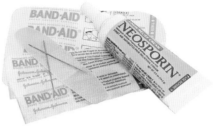

BUNIONS

A bunion is a bony bump at the base of your big toe (caused by your first metatarsal bone turning outward, pointing your big toe inward), right at the joint connecting your big toe to your foot. Bunions can be red and painful. Outside surgery, your best bet is to make sure that your forefoot has plenty of room by purchasing shoes with wide toe boxes. You'll want to avoid narrow shoes and high heels. You can train with a bunion as long as the pain doesn't force you into an unnatural stride and the pressure doesn't result in severe inflammation of the bursa that surround the joint.

CALF STRAIN

Calf strains cause pain and tightness in your calves, usually following intense exercise, such as running repetitions, hill repeats, drills, or heavy resistance training. With minor pain, you can move straight into the following exercises. If the strain makes it hard to walk (and impossible to run), you'll need to take a few days off to allow healing. If you're susceptible to calf strains, you'll want to include both of the following exercises in your post-run routine (two to three times per week).

Rope stretch

This stretch helps to relieve tightness in your calves post-run, leaving you less susceptible to lingering pain and stiffness.

Lie on your back with one knee bent, foot flat on the floor, and with the other leg raised and straightened. Loop the rope around the ball of your foot. Gently pull your toes and the ball of your foot toward your shin while *simultaneously* tightening (flexing) your raised quadriceps muscle (front thigh). Hold for 30 seconds, then repeat with the opposite leg.

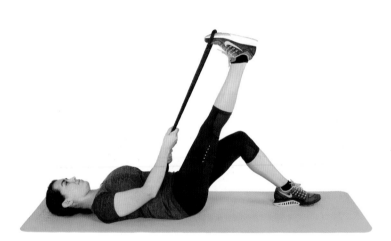

Heel raises – straight knee

Straight knee heel raises help strengthen your calves through a full range of motion.

1 Place the balls of your feet on a platform, feet hip-width apart, with your heels hanging off the platform. Use a chair or other support for balance. First, lower your heels so that they drop beneath the edge of the platform (don't overstretch!).

2 Next, raise your heels as high as you can, coming up on your toes. Pause at the top for 1–2 seconds, then return to your starting position. Repeat 10–15 times.

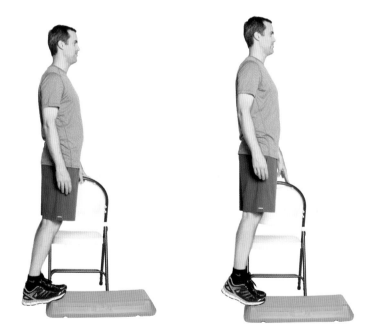

CHAFING

Chafing refers to painful irritation that results when you have skin rubbing against skin (e.g., your inner thighs during a run) or skin rubbing against certain fabrics (e.g., nipples rubbing against a loose shirt, causing "runner's nipple," in which the nipples are rubbed so raw that they often bleed). The best way to combat chafing is to apply products (e.g., Body Glide) that reduce friction without staining your clothes. Lubricants like petroleum jelly also work, but staining will be an issue. For inner-thigh chafing, you can opt for half tights, tights, or long shorts to prevent skin-on-skin rubbing. Post-run, apply an antibiotic ointment to speed healing and prevent infection. Unless the pain is unbearable, there's no reason you can't run.

DELAYED ONSET MUSCLE SORENESS (DOMS)

DOMS is muscular soreness that runners experience in the days following excessive exercise. Pain usually peaks forty-eight to seventy-two hours after the exercise bout. DOMS is thought to be caused by eccentric muscle contractions (contractions that occur when the muscle must contract and stretch simultaneously, as happens when your foot touches down during a running stride, simultaneously contracting and lengthening your quadriceps muscles). Recently, researchers have also proposed that there's a nervous system component to the syndrome. For immediate relief of symptoms, try icing, a cold bath, massage, or anti-inflammatories. If all else fails, try complete rest. Symptoms disappear within five to seven days, and episodes of DOMS usually immunize runners against repeat episodes (for at least a few weeks). If you have pain but normal muscular range of motion, you can try the following easy recovery activity.

Easy Distance Run

The best remedy might be limiting your next workout to easy walking or an easy-effort distance run. Keep it short. Keep it slow. And don't extend your stride beyond what feels (relatively) comfortable.

GROIN STRAIN

Groin strains occur when you strain any of five adductor muscles (muscles that pull your leg inward toward the midline of your body) or damage the associated connective tissue. Pain will be felt in the groin or inner thigh area, especially when lifting your knee, and it can come on suddenly or gradually. You can usually train through mild groin pain (although you may need a reduced workload). If the pain is severe, you'll need to see a health professional to rule out a sports hernia or some other severe muscular or connective tissue damage. To help prevent groin strains or to limit the recurrence of strains once your injury has healed, try the following exercises.

Hip adduction

This exercise strengthens your hip adductors and keeps your hips stable through your full stride and during foot strike.

1 Secure a resistance band to an anchor or stationary object at ankle level. While standing, loop the band around your anchor-side leg, just above the ankle, with your other foot positioned slightly back (so that it's not in the way). Hold on to a chair or other support for balance.

2 Keeping your leg straight, pull your leg inward, in front of and across your other leg. Slowly return to the start position and repeat for 5–10 repetitions. Switch legs and repeat.

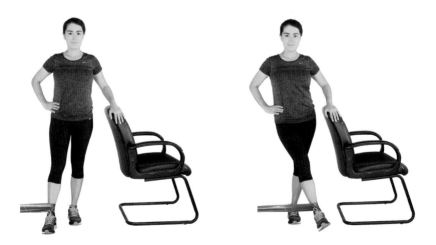

Leg lifts

Leg lifts strengthen your lower abdominals, aiding core stability and knee lift.

1 Lie on your back with your knees bent, your heels on the floor, your hands behind your head, and your head lifted slightly off the floor.

2 Keeping the bend in your knees, raise your feet to about 45°. Then lower your legs until your heels almost touch the floor. Start with 10–15 repetitions, and gradually build up to between 40 and 50 reps.

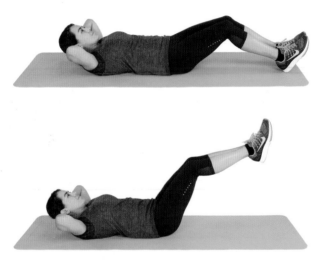

Leg swings

Leg swings are a form of dynamic stretching that can help activate your core and create a better range of motion in your hip flexors, hip abductors, and hip adductors. Many runners include leg swings as part of their warm-up routine.

1 Begin with forward and backward leg swings. Balance against a wall, hold on to a chair, or use some other support.

2 Standing tall, swing your leg (on the same side as your supporting hand) forward and backward at the hip, allowing your swinging leg to bend slightly at the knee, for 10 or more repetitions.

3 Next, use both hands to support yourself while facing the wall, chair, or other support, then lean slightly forward while swinging your leg across your body, keeping your upper body mostly motionless and pointing your toes upward as you swing.

4 Then swing your leg back the other way, pulling the leg as high as it will go, for a total of 10 or more repetitions.

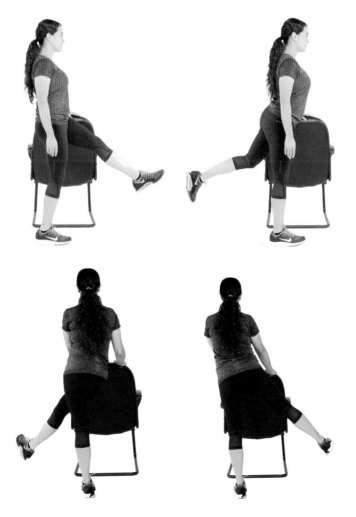

HAMSTRING STRAIN

Hamstring strains cause pain and tightness in your hamstrings (your rear thigh muscles) that can restrict your movement. With mild hamstring strains, you can sometimes continue training with reduced volume, but understand that hamstring injuries have a tendency to become chronic; a majority of runners who suffer hamstring strains will become reinjured within a year. In other words, you might be better served taking a week off rather than risking long-term injury. Severe hamstring injuries will absolutely require time off (from a few weeks to a few months). Rushing your return to training will only lead to reinjury—and hamstrings, when they reinjure, tend to reinjure completely. Icing and anti-inflammatories can help with pain management. And the following exercises can help to prevent or, when you're ready, rehabilitate hamstring injuries.

Single-leg deadlifts

This is a great exercise for strengthening your hamstrings (and glutes) while simultaneously increasing your range of motion. It also improves balance and stability.

1 Start from a standing position, feet hip-width apart. I'd recommend using a chair or other support for balance.

2 Keeping your spine straight, bend forward at the hips while lifting the leg closest to your chair (or other support) straight behind you (it's OK for both your knees to bend slightly) and reaching with your free hand toward the ground. If not using a support, reach with both hands toward the ground. Then return to your starting position. Do 5–10 repetitions, then switch legs.

3 As you improve at this exercise, add weight by holding a dumbbell.

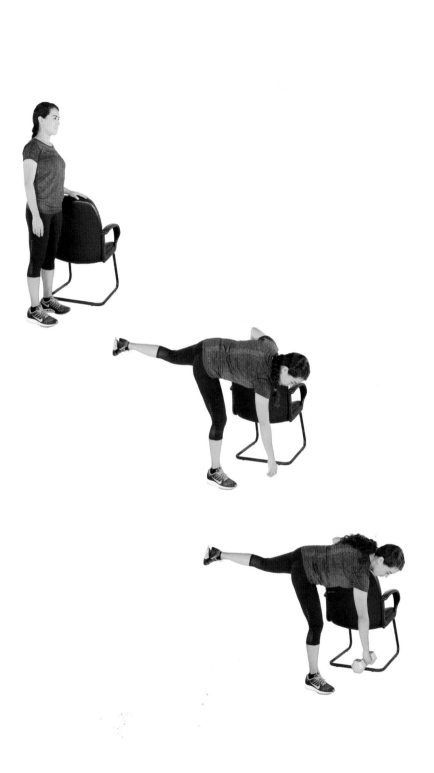

AIS hamstrings

This stretching exercise increases the range of motion for your hamstrings.

1 Lie on your back, bend your non-stretching leg (foot flat on the floor), and loop your rope around the arch of your foot (exercising leg), with that leg extended flat on the floor.

2 Lift your exercising leg off the floor, using your thigh and hip-flexor muscles, while keeping your hips on the floor. When you can't lift your leg any higher, use the rope to increase the stretch a tiny bit more (never beyond your natural range of motion). Don't hold the stretch. Instead, immediately return your leg to the start position. Do 10 repetitions, then switch legs.

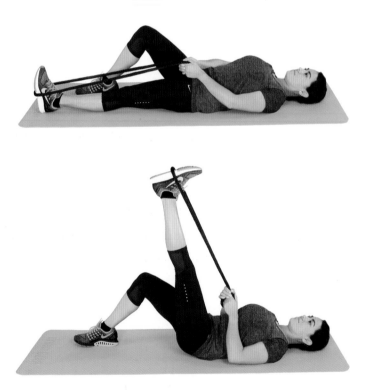

HEAT ILLNESS

Heat illnesses can include heat cramps, heat exhaustion, and heat stroke. All result from overheating due to high temperatures, high humidity, or hard training. *Heat exhaustion* will produce the following symptoms: cramps, nausea, headache, and general weakness. Since heat exhaustion can progress to heat stroke, it's important that you stop training, get in a cool environment, and rehydrate. *Heat stroke* is a life-threatening condition caused by prolonged exposure to extreme heat and/or humidity, as well as by exercising in those extreme conditions. It can cause damage to the brain and other organs, as well as leading to shock or even death. Symptoms include:

→ Fever greater than 104°F

→ Dry, hot, red skin

→ Confusion

→ Rapid, weak pulse

→ Seizures

→ Unconsciousness

For heat stroke, according to the National Institutes of Health:

→ Have the person lie down in a cool place with his or her feet lifted 12 inches

→ Call 911 immediately

→ Apply cool, wet cloths to the person's skin

→ If the person is conscious and alert, offer a sports drink or salted beverage (1 teaspoon of salt per quart) to sip

HEAVY LEGS

Heavy legs syndrome often results from training too hard, either during a single workout or over the course of several workouts. Your legs will feel heavy and unresponsive. Your energy levels will be low. Your motivation will be sapped. The best recovery plan is to schedule a series of long, easy distance runs—the easier the better. Another approach that sometimes works is to increase carbohydrate and fluid intake for a few days; this rebuilds your muscle glycogen stores and rehydrates your body (both potential factors in heavy legs).

HIP PAIN

You might experience nonspecific pain in your hip area. Unless you experience sharp pain, icing isn't advised, as hip pain often radiates, making it hard to pinpoint the specific origin. The decision to run or not run should be based upon the level of pain—if it's mild, you can train with reduced volume and intensity; if it's severe, better to take a few days off. For injury prevention and rehab once the injury has healed, try the exercises that follow. You might also consider the hip adduction exercises from the groin strain entry and the lunge walk and side steps exercises from the IT band syndrome entry.

Hip flexors stretch

This simple stretch loosens your hip flexors (the muscles at the front of the hip that move your knee toward your chest).

1 Kneel with your left knee forward. With your hands on your hips, move forward by shifting your hips forward (not by bending at the waist); this increases the stretch on your hip flexors. Hold for 30 seconds, then switch legs.

2 As long as you're already in this position, you might as well take the opportunity to stretch your quadriceps (front thigh muscles). Grab your trailing foot and lift upward until you feel the stretch on your quadriceps. At this point, you have the option of moving your hips

forward to increase the stretch on your hip flexors. Hold for 30 seconds. Then switch legs and repeat.

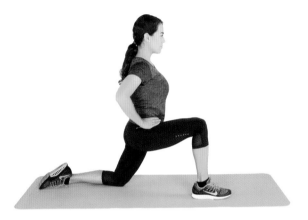

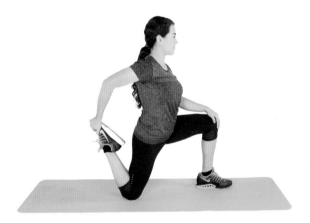

Monster walk

Monster walking works your hip flexors, hip extensors, and hip abductors, providing a terrific all-around strengthening workout for your hips.

1 Loop a resistance band or resistance tubing around your ankles (or for less resistance, right above or below your knees), bend your knees slightly, feet hip-width apart, with arms either hanging loosely at your sides or with your hands on your hips.

2 Step forward and to the side at a 45° angle, keeping the bend in your knees. Step forward and to the opposite side at a 45° angle. Take 10 to 20 steps. Start with 1 set and work up to 2–3 sets.

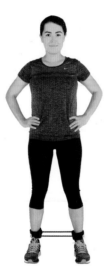 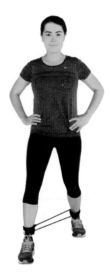

IT BAND SYNDROME

Your iliotibial (IT) band is a thick cord of connective tissue that runs along the outside of your leg, from your hip to your knee. IT band syndrome is usually felt as sharp pain on the outside of your knee, but it can also cause pain on the outside of your hip—on the bony prominence at the top of your thigh bone (femur). IT band syndrome has been attributed to both overuse (repeating the same physical motion, as occurs during distance running) and to weak hip and glute (butt) muscles. Barring preventative exercises or treatment, it can progress to an injury requiring weeks (or months) of non-running. Unless you're immobilized by pain, you can train—unlike other injuries, you might do best by including your normal variety of training, rather than limiting yourself to easy running (since this is often an overuse injury, performing the same running stride over and over can make the injury worse). If your pain is mild, there's no reason you can't start including the exercises below in your strength program (if your pain increases, of course, you'll need to discontinue the exercises). For this injury, prevention is the best cure. In the meantime, icing and anti-inflammatories can provide temporary relief from the pain.

Side steps

Side steps will strengthen and stabilize your hip abductors.

1 Loop the resistance band or tubing around your ankles (or for less resistance, right above or below your knees). Bend your knees slightly with your feet hip-width apart.

2 Step directly to the side with one foot until the band provides significant resistance. Then slide your other foot over to re-create your original stance. Repeat 5–10 times in one direction, and then reverse direction for 5–10 more repetitions.

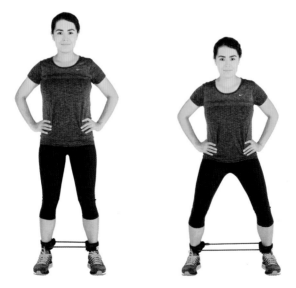

Lunge walk

The lunge walk will strengthen your hips and glutes, improving your stability during runs.

1 Start from a standing position with your arms hanging at your sides.

2 Take a step forward, bending at the knee until your thigh is parallel to the ground. Your front knee should be lined up over your front foot (but not ahead of it!). Now step forward into another lunge with the opposite leg (obviously, you'll have to rise up as you step forward). Start with 5–10 steps, then gradually increase to between 20 and 30 steps (don't overdo this one!).

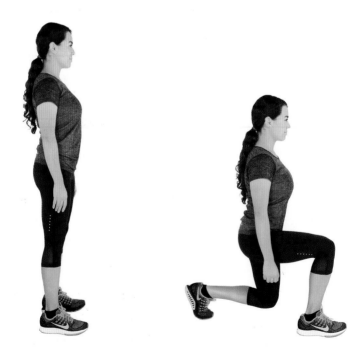

IT band stretch

This stretch is only advised for people who are flexible (i.e., who can get into the position without discomfort).

Sit on the floor with one leg extended in front of you, and with your other leg folded back, your foot tucked next to your hip. Your knees should be 1–2 inches apart, your thighs almost parallel. Reach toward your toes while bringing your head over the straightened knee. You should feel the "pull" along the outside of your stretched leg. Hold for 30–60 seconds, then repeat with the opposite leg.

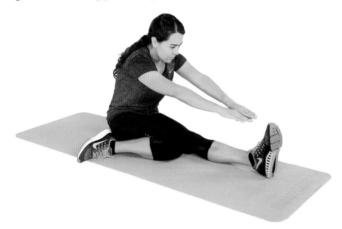

KNEE PAIN (GENERAL)

Generalized, sharp knee pain can occur on the front of the knee without an obvious inciting incident or structural impairment (i.e., there will be no visible swelling or damage). This pain is hard to diagnose and might result from damage to pain nerves themselves (through poor running mechanics). As with most other injuries, the decision about whether to train should be based on the level of pain you're experiencing. The following exercises will strengthen muscles that help stabilize the knee, making them advisable for injury prevention and a must during rehabilitation once the pain has receded. Aside from the following exercises, consider performing the lunge walk from the entry for IT band syndrome.

Step-ups

Step-ups strengthen your quadriceps and glutes, helping to stabilize your stride.

1 Stand in front of a raised platform.

2 Step onto the platform, making sure that your entire foot is on the platform. Your platform shouldn't be so high that your knee exceeds a 90° bend.

3 Rise up onto the platform, generating force with your forward (bent) leg. Use your opposite leg for balance only, letting it come to rest lightly on the platform. Do 5–10 reps, then switch legs. As you get stronger, you can add weight by holding dumbbells.

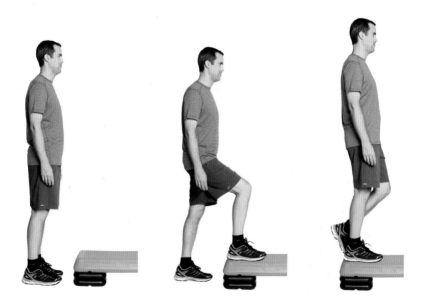

Step-downs

This exercise builds stability in the hips and knees, and it's great for preventing and rehabbing knee injuries.

1 Balance on one foot at the edge of a raised platform. Feel free to use a chair or other support for balance. Hold your other foot out in front of the platform, with that knee slightly bent.

2 Lower your hips by bending the knee of your weight-bearing leg. Your free leg/foot will drop as you lower your hips—as if you're "stepping down." To avoid injury, make sure the knee and foot of your weight-bearing leg remain aligned. Rise to your starting position. Do 5–10 reps with each leg.

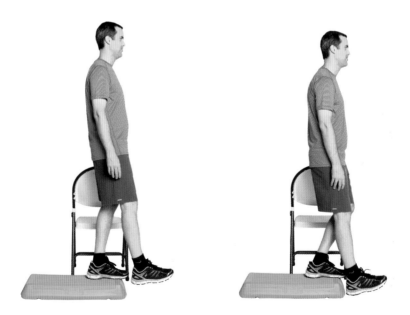

LOWER BACK PAIN & STIFFNESS

Pain and stiffness in your lower back can affect your running stride and make it difficult to perform everyday activities. While this condition can result from spinal problems (e.g., a bulging disc) or sciatica, it's often caused by lower back muscles that are in spasm (and won't release). If pain and stiffness are mild, you're probably OK to run easy distance. If pain and tightness are severe, you should see a health professional to rule out a spinal injury or sciatica.

The daydreamer

This position helps relieve tension in your lower back (when muscle spasms are the cause) in just a few minutes.

Lie on your back with your arms out to your sides, hands at approximately waist level, with your lower legs and feet propped on a chair. Keep a 90° bend in your knees and try to position your feet so that they don't roll outward. Take slow, deep breaths. Relax in this position for 5–10 minutes.

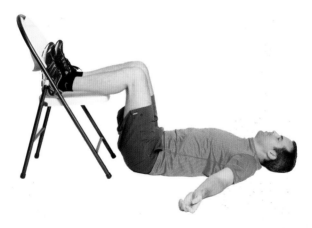

Knee to chest

This traditional stretch helps relieve tension in your lower back.

1 Lie on your back, one leg bent at the knee, foot down. Grasp your opposite leg at the knee and lift it toward your chest, keeping your hips on the floor. Don't overstretch.

2 If you're flexible, repeat the above instructions with your down leg flat on the floor.

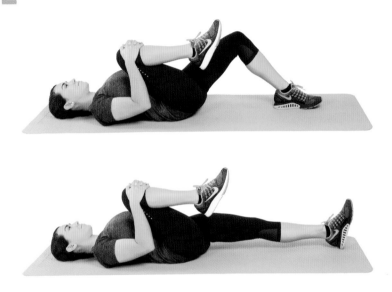

MENISCUS TEAR

Your lateral and medial menisci are two pads of fibrocartilage that provide shock absorption and structural support for your knee. Damage to your meniscus is felt as pain at the side or center of your knee, accompanied by swelling and usually following a twisting motion. Symptoms can include a popping sensation at the time of the injury, swelling that gets worse, or, in the aftermath of the injury, the feeling that your knee is "catching" or otherwise unstable. For this injury, you'll need to see a health professional—and stop running until you do.

MUSCLE CRAMPS—HAMSTRINGS & CALVES

These are sudden, involuntary, and sustained muscle contractions that cause pain. Static stretching is an effective, immediate, traditional remedy for hamstring and calf cramps (illustrated below). A quicker remedy (but hard for many less-flexible runners to perform) is "weight-bearing ankle dorsiflexion," which is a confusing way of saying that you should stand, then reach down and pull up your same-side toes of the leg that is cramping. You *must* stop running until the cramp is relieved. Once it's gone, you can exercise as long as you limit both volume and intensity.

Hamstring static stretch

A traditional hamstring static stretch should relieve your cramp pronto.

While sitting tall on the floor, extend one leg in front of you and fold the other with the bottom of your foot pressed against the opposite inner thigh. Bend forward from the waist without hunching your back and reach toward your toes. Don't overstretch! When you reach the end of your range of motion, hold until the cramp releases (hold up to a maximum of 60 seconds—if the cramp persists, release the stretch for a few seconds and then try again).

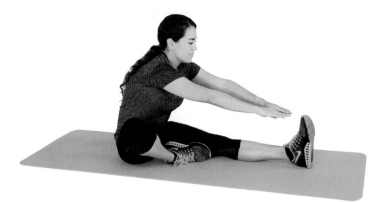

Calf static stretch

While there are many different static stretches for the calves, this is the quickest and easiest to perform when a cramp strikes.

Put your hands shoulder height and palms flat against a wall or other support. Step back with one leg. Bend the knee of the front leg while keeping the back leg straight. Move forward at the hips while keeping your back heel firmly planted on the ground. When you reach your full range of motion, hold until the cramp releases (hold up to a maximum of 60 seconds—if the cramp persists, release the stretch for a few seconds and then try again).

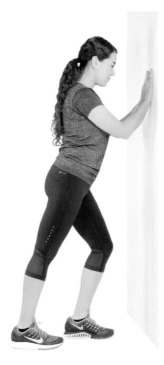

OSTEOARTHRITIS

Osteoarthritis causes pain, swelling, and immobility in a joint, and it occurs when your articular cartilage (the cartilage that provides the smooth coating on the surface ends of bones) becomes thin; this narrows the joint space, sometimes to the point of bone-on-bone contact. Most osteoarthritis is genetic, with age and trauma as additional factors. Running doesn't cause it, but there's an indication that running can help prevent or delay its onset. Masters runners should consider getting an X-ray to check on their cartilage thickness; that way, if thinning has occurred, you can make informed training choices. A post-run strengthening routine can keep your hips and knees tracking more efficiently, possibly reducing symptoms. If you suspect you have osteoarthritis, you should consult a health professional.

PIRIFORMIS SYNDROME

Your piriformis muscle is located slightly above the center-middle portion of your glutes (butt), immediately adjacent to the sciatic nerve (see "Sciatica" in this section). Sharp pain, tingling, or numbness in this area is usually related to pressure on the sciatic nerve, but it can also originate from the piriformis muscle itself—if the muscle is irritated, the nerve tends to be irritated. As long as pain allows, you can continue running. But you should implement the following exercises.

Knee to opposite shoulder

This stretch should relieve tension in the piriformis.

Lie on your back, one leg flat on the floor. Grasp your opposite leg at the knee and lift it toward your opposite shoulder, keeping your hips on the floor. Don't overstretch.

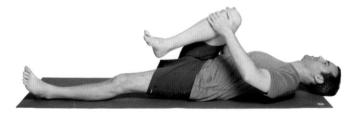

The clam

Doing the clam should strengthen the piriformis and other muscles involved in hip abduction and rotation.

1 Lie on your side with your legs stacked one on top of the other, and your knees bent at about 45°.

2 Lift your top knee while keeping your feet stacked. Then close your legs. Repeat 10–15 times with each leg. To increase resistance, loop a resistance band just above your knees.

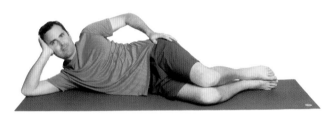

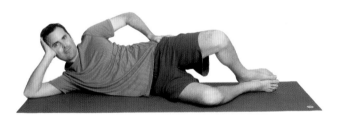

PLANTAR FASCIITIS (PF)

Plantar fasciitis (the bane of masters runners) can be felt at the point where the heel meets the arch (press on the inside of your arch, against the heel, and you'll probably scream if you have PF). That said, pain from PF can radiate, and many runners mistakenly identify the first sign of PF as a heel bruise. Pain might also be felt along the arch or elsewhere in your foot. PF can stop your running in its tracks, then linger for months or even years. The onset can be sudden, with an inciting incident (like stepping wrong on a rock), or it can develop gradually, over weeks or months (often, in the latter case, the cause is thought to be injured or weakened muscles in the foot rather than injury to the PF itself). In the case of sudden onset, you'll have to stop running—*immediately*—until the injury heals. For PF that develops gradually, you'll probably be able to continue running during the early stages of the injury. At some point, however, PF tends to progress to a point where running becomes impossible. That's why you'll want to start injury prevention exercises at the very first hint of pain.

Towel toe curls

This is the simplest exercise for staving off plantar fasciitis. It strengthens the intrinsic muscles of your feet.

Sit barefoot in a chair with a towel spread on the floor in front of you. Put a shoe on the towel's opposite end to create minor resistance. While keeping your heels on the floor, pull the towel toward you by scrunching your toes. Bunch the towel beneath your arch (or behind your heels) until you've reeled in its full length. Do this 1–3 times.

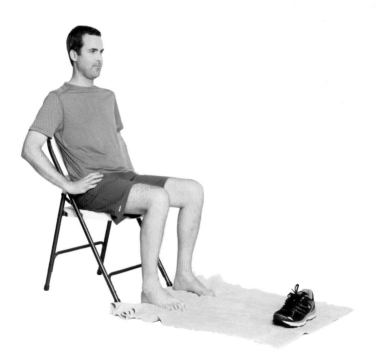

Big-toe taps

This exercise helps strengthen the muscles that control extension and flexion of your toes, which, when strong, help reduce pressure on the plantar fascia.

1 Stand barefoot with your feet hip-width apart. Lift your big toes as you simultaneously press down with the other four toes of each foot.

2 Now reverse what you're doing. Press down with your big toes as you raise your remaining toes. Start with 5–10 reps, then increase to 15–20 reps. (And be prepared for it to take a couple of tries before you get the coordination down for this exercise.)

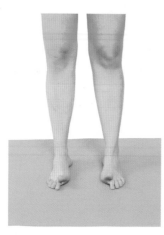 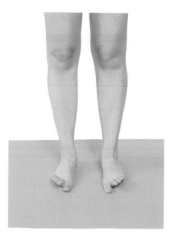

Superfeet Arch Supports

Some runners get temporary relief from Superfeet Arch Supports (especially while walking), although I'd recommend against making this a permanent solution, as developing a stronger and properly functioning arch *without artificial support* is key to avoiding and beating this injury.

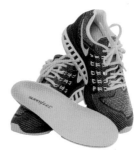

Insert the Superfeet Arch Supports into your running shoes.

QUADRICEPS PAIN

Sometimes, runners find themselves with achy, painful quadriceps (front thigh) muscles and no idea how it happened—no specific mistake they can put their finger on. Untreated, this pain can become chronic. And it can become intense enough to make running torture. Even walking up and down stairs can become pure agony. Besides some of the quad-strengthening exercises we've already introduced (e.g., step-ups from the knee pain entry and lunge walk from the IT band syndrome entry), the following exercise has proved effective.

Downhill running

Downhill running increases the workload on your front thighs (quadriceps), triggering greater strength adaptations in the muscles. But you need to be careful with downhill running. A few years back, in an article that appeared in both *Running Times* and *Runner's World* (same parent company), I recommended downhill running as a cure for chronic quadriceps pain. I'd personally had such a severe case of quad pain before the 2005 national cross country championships that I'd considered withdrawing. In desperation, I'd jogged up a local mountain, then charged a two-mile downhill run, hoping to trigger overcompensation (increased strengthening in the quads). It worked. The soreness cleared up, and a week later I won the masters national championship. In the article, I suggested that runners start with some short downhill strides, then build up to a longer downhill run. Unfortunately, one reader decided to copy my two-mile downhill charge. "Now I can't walk," she wrote in an email. By skipping the downhill strides, she left her body unprepared for the longer downhill run. There was nothing I could do for her. But there's something I can do for you: "Start with strides!"

DOWNHILL STRIDES: After warming up, run 4 downhill strides (10–15 seconds) at about an 85 percent effort. Walk back to the start for recovery. Add 2 strides to each successive workout until you reach a maximum of 8 strides.

DOWNHILL CONTINUOUS RUNNING: Once you can complete 8 downhill strides, try 3 minutes of downhill running at tempo effort. Add 1–2 minutes to successive workouts until you reach a maximum of 12 minutes.

RUNNER'S KNEE (AKA PATELLOFEMORAL PAIN SYNDROME OR CHONDROMALACIA)

This is the most common running injury, accounting for up to one third of reported injuries every year. If you've got runner's knee, you'll feel pain behind or around your kneecap, and there might be a popping or crackling sensation in the knee. It's caused by irritation of the cartilage in your kneecap joint. This can be a biomechanical issue, or it can result from trauma to the kneecap. Your best bet for combatting runner's knee is to prevent it. And the best way to do that is to perform the Beginner's Body Strengthening routine on page 275, since strong quadriceps muscles, hips, and hamstrings are essential for smooth patella (kneecap) tracking. You might also consider including the monster walk from the entry on hip pain and step-downs from the entry on knee pain. If you experience runner's knee, cut back on your mileage and try to avoid excessive bending or loading at the joint (e.g., squatting). Anti-inflammatories can help with the pain and inflammation. If the condition persists, you'll want to see a health professional.

SCIATICA

Your sciatic nerve runs from each side of your lower spine through the center of your glutes (buttocks), down your hamstrings, and all the way to your feet. It's the biggest nerve in your body. And when you feel pain—from a herniated disc or irritated piriformis muscle or some other cause—it's known as "sciatica." Runners will feel pain, tingling (pins and needles), and/or numbness in one or all of the following areas: lower back, buttocks, hamstrings, calves, and feet. For many runners, chiropractic treatment provides relief. Others have found success with core-muscle and stability-exercise programs designed by physical therapists. Since complete rest isn't always effective, try the following three exercises if you're experiencing symptoms.

Knees to chest

This simple stretch can reduce tension on your lower back and pelvis.

Lie on your back with your knees bent, feet flat on the floor. Now, gently grasp your knees with your hands and bring them slowly toward your chest (for your first time, you might want to bring your knees to your chest one at a time, as this will put less sudden pressure on your back and abdominal muscles). Relax while you gently hug your knees toward your chest. Only hold this stretch for a few seconds, then return to your start position. Repeat 5–10 times.

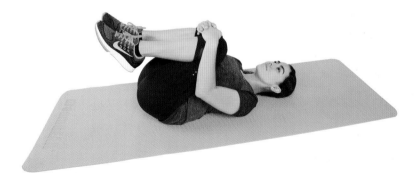

Cobra stretch

This stretch works well if you have a herniated disc and *if you're young.* Older runners might have trouble with the flexibility required for this stretch.

1 Lie facedown on the floor, feet hip-width apart, palms next to your shoulders.

2 Inhale as you straighten your arms and slowly lift your upper torso and head, keeping your pelvis on the floor. Only go as far as is comfortable, then slowly return to your starting position. Start with 3–5 reps and build up to 10–15.

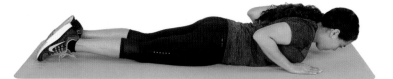

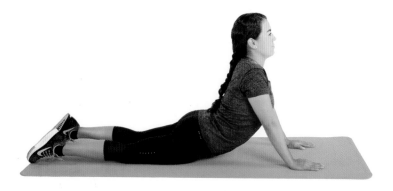

Ankle pumps with hamstring stretch

Here's one final exercise to stretch the sciatic nerve, helping it to move through the tight tissue that surrounds it.

1 Lie on your back, one leg bent with the foot flat on the floor. Lift your other leg, grasping behind the knee (it's OK for the knee to be slightly bent) until you reach your full range of motion.

2 Pump the ankle by moving it forward and backward, like you're working a gas pedal. Start with 10 reps for each leg, then gradually increase to 30, performing about one ankle pump per second. As you become more skilled at this exercise, you can create a true glide of the sciatic nerve by lifting your head and neck up (flexion) as you point your toes away from you (plantarflexion), and then lowering your head and neck back down (extension) as you pull your toes upward toward your head/neck (dorsiflexion).

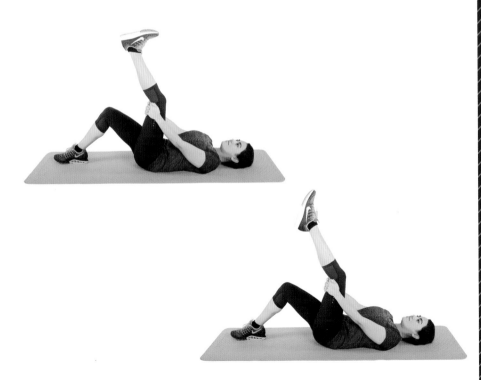

SHIN SPLINTS — FRONT

With front shin splints, you'll feel sharp pain along the outside of your shin(s). Continued training will be determined by your level of pain (i.e., it's up to you). Icing and anti-inflammatories can provide temporary relief. Besides the following exercises, the wobble board exercises from the ankle sprain entry are very effective for preventing and rehabbing this injury.

Seated toe-taps

These directly strengthen the muscles on the front of your shins.

1 Sit in a chair with your legs bent 90° at your knees, feet flat on the floor.

2 Quickly lift and lower your feet without raising your heels, until you feel a "burn" in the muscles on the front of your shins, which could take from a few seconds to 2–3 minutes (the entire time counts as one set). Start with 1 set and build to 2 or more.

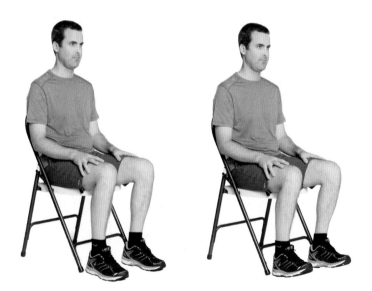

Ankle dorsiflexion

This is a more intense version of the strengthening from seated toe-taps.

1 Sit on the floor with one leg extended in front of you, the other leg bent at the knee. Attach a resistance band around the top of your foot (extended leg) and anchor it to a secure object. Put your hands behind you, palms down, for support. Start with your foot angled forward.

2 Pull your foot back toward your shin. When you can't pull it any farther back, slowly return your foot to its starting position. Do 5–10 reps with each foot.

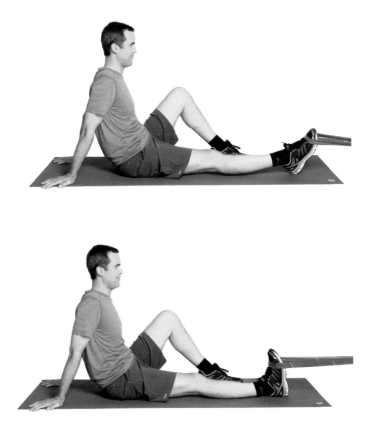

SHIN SPLINTS — MEDIAL

With medial shin splints (also known as "medial tibial stress syndrome"), you'll feel sharp pain along the inside of your shin(s). You can usually run through the early stages of medial shin splints, but be fore-warned that this injury tends to worsen, often to the point where running becomes impossible (in worst-case scenarios, this syndrome is a precursor to a stress fracture). You'll want to start injury-prevention exercises at the very first inkling of pain.

Ankle inversion

This is the best exercise for both preventing and treating medial shin splints.

1 Sit in a chair with one end of a resistance band secured to an anchor (or other secure object) at ankle level. Loop the band's other end around the arch side (inside) of your foot.

2 Keep your knee facing forward and your heel on the floor as you pull your foot inward (i.e., limit motion to your lower leg). When your foot reaches its maximum range of motion, slowly return to your starting position. Do 5–10 reps with each foot.

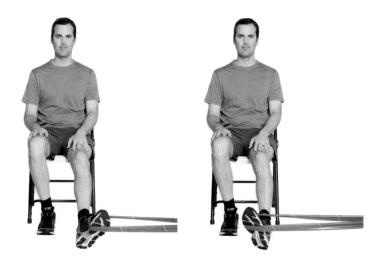

Ankle plantarflexion

This is another good exercise for preventing and treating medial shin splints.

1   Sit on the floor with one leg extended in front of you, the other bent at the knee. Loop a resistance band around your foot (extended leg) and apply pressure against the bottom of your foot by pulling the band toward your torso.

2   Push your foot forward—holding the band taut to provide resistance—until you reach your maximum range of motion, then slowly return to your starting position. Do 5–10 reps with each foot.

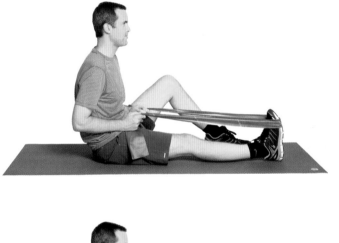

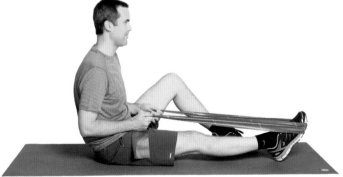

SIDE STITCH

A side stitch is a sharp pain that runners generally feel just beneath their rib cage (usually on the right side, but it can occur on the left as well—and also less frequently in other regions of the abdomen). Far from a minor ache, a side stitch can be completely crippling when it occurs during a training run or a race. While the cause of side stitches has yet to be definitely determined, several theories have emerged. For a long while, the operating theory was that stitches were the result of a spasm of the diaphragm. Recently, a new culprit has emerged: irritation of the parietal peritoneum; this occurs when core muscles grow tired, causing back muscles to exert pressure on nerves that cause pain in the abdomen and side. Less-credible theories put the blame on breathing patterns, diet, dehydration, and fitness. My personal favorite trick for combating side stitches (not illustrated) is four-step breathing: First, inhale twice in succession (without exhaling), taking the two breaths in sync with two strides and filling your lungs to maximum capacity; next, purse your lips and blow out intensely for two more strides; repeat for thirty to sixty seconds. Four-step breathing helps relieve the tension (regardless of origin) that fuels stitches.

Hold side, bend side-to-side, bend forward, and deep-breathe

You'll often see runners performing a mix of these exercises to provide relief from a stitch.

1 First, with your hands on your hips, bend sideways away from the side of the stitch. Hold for a few seconds.

2 Next, try bending forward while grabbing your side (pinching the point of the stitch between thumb and fingers). Hold for a few seconds. While you're trying these exercises, practice deep breathing: Take slow, deep breaths, inhaling and exhaling fully.

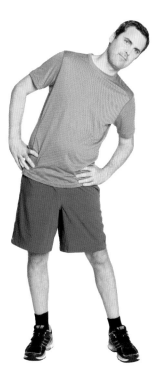

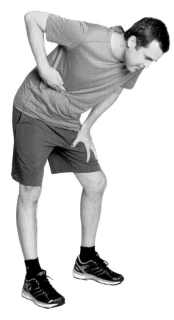

Core work

Since a fatiguing core is thought to be behind stitches, it can't hurt to add a couple of core exercises to those you'll already be doing as part of your post-run routine.

1   Start with a set of "bird dogs." Get on all fours, with your spine straight through your neck and head.

2   Lift one arm and the opposite leg, extending the leg straight back and reaching forward with your open palm. Hold for 5–10 seconds, then repeat 5–10 times (or as fitness dictates).

3   Next up is a "side bridge." Begin by lying on your side, resting on your forearm, hip, knee, and foot with your legs stacked, your other hand on your hip.

4   Lift your hips from the floor until your spine is straightened, with your weight on your forearm and feet. Hold for 5–10 seconds, then repeat 5–10 times (or as fitness dictates).

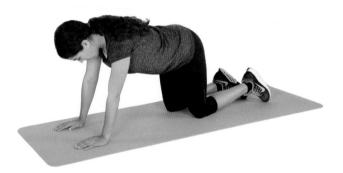

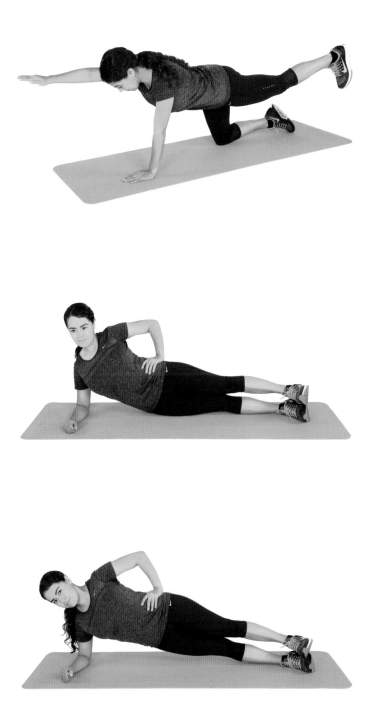

STRESS FRACTURE

Stress fractures are tiny cracks in bone. Runners are especially susceptible to them during periods of increased training intensity and volume
(e.g., at the very beginning of new running programs). During these periods, your body digs out tiny pockets of old, weak bone so that you can
replace it with newer, stronger bone, leaving you with porous bone that's
more likely to fracture. (This is a good reason to schedule only incremental increases in training!) If you suspect that you have a stress fracture,
you should see a podiatrist, orthopedist, or other health professional.
Stress fractures most frequently occur in the feet (metatarsals) and the
lower leg (tibia), but they can also occur in the femur, pelvis, and any-
place where training puts excessive stress on bone. You'll have to stop
running while the fracture heals—and be prepared for a walking boot or
cast.

BEGINNER'S BODY STRENGTHENING

BEGINNING THE SECOND OR THIRD WEEK of your program, you can start to incorporate sessions of resistance training into your weekly schedule. Start with two sessions, and then only add a third session if your schedule allows (i.e., if you're not too fatigued from the running and resistance training you're already doing). As your running volume increases, you may choose to scale back on the number of strength sessions per week, with competitive runners performing only a single session per week. For your initial sessions, you should include the following eight exercises. You'll also find an additional nine exercises listed (along with page numbers for photo instruction); after you're comfortable with the initial exercises, you can add these additional exercises to your routine—one or two exercises at a time. Five quick guidelines:

1 Start with no more than a single set of each exercise for your first week of training (some runners will stay at 1 set for several weeks). After that, you can add 1 set per week, up to a maximum of 3 sets. Never add sets if you're sore from the previous workout.

2 Add free weights (e.g., dumbbells and barbells) to exercises when a session including 3 sets becomes too easy.

3 Never do resistance training on consecutive days; you need at least 1 recovery day between sessions.

4 Allow 2–3 minutes between sets.

5 Perform resistance training after running, not before. Or you can do your resistance training at a different time of the day than your running.

Always remember that, as a runner, your resistance-training goals are governed by a commitment to all-around strength. You aren't a body-builder, and you aren't an Olympic power lifter. Don't train to exhaustion. A moderate effort level will produce the best results.

Note: Some of the following exercises also appear in the injury-prevention exercises photo instruction. In those instances, the photo instruction is being reproduced here.

BEGINNER'S BODY STRENGTHENING—ESSENTIAL ROUTINE

The following eight exercises should be included in the initial routines of all runners.

Air squat

Air squats strengthen your quadriceps, hamstrings, and glutes.

1 Stand straight with your feet hip-width apart, arms straight out from your shoulders. Your toes should be pointed slightly out (this keeps pressure off your knees during the squat and also helps prevent your knees from angling inward).

2 Bend your knees, pushing your hips back until your thighs are parallel to the floor. Simultaneously bring your arms forward; this helps you to maintain balance. Push upward with your quadriceps (front thighs) to return to your starting position. Start with 5 reps, then build up to 10–12.

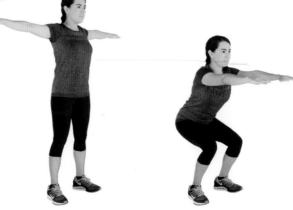

Step-ups

Step-ups strengthen your quadriceps and glutes.

1 Stand in front of a raised platform.

2 Step onto the platform, making sure that your entire foot is on the platform. Your platform shouldn't be so high that your knee exceeds a 90° bend.

3 Rise up onto the platform, generating force with your forward (bent) leg. Use your opposite leg for balance only, letting it come to rest lightly on the platform. Do 5–10 reps, then switch legs. As you get stronger, you can add weight by holding dumbbells.

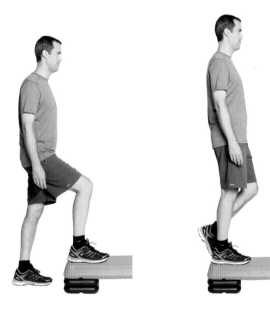

Single-leg deadlifts

This is a great exercise for strengthening your hamstrings (and glutes) while simultaneously increasing your range of motion. It also improves balance and stability.

1 Start from a standing position, feet hip-width apart. I'd recommend using a chair or other support for balance.

2 Keeping your spine straight, bend forward at the hips while lifting the leg closest to your chair (or other support) straight behind you (it's OK for both your knees to bend slightly) and reaching with your free hand toward the ground. If you're not using a support, reach with both hands toward the ground. Then return to your starting position. Do 5–10 repetitions, then switch legs.

3 As you improve at this exercise, add weight by holding a dumbbell.

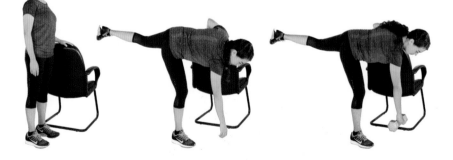

Side leg lifts

Side leg lifts work your hip abductors.

1 Lie on your side with your legs stacked. Rest your head on your arm, and keep your shoulders, hips, and feet in a line.

2 Lift your top leg to 45° in a smooth motion, then bring it back down. Do 10–15 reps with each leg.

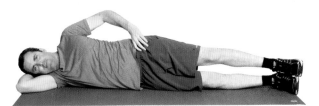

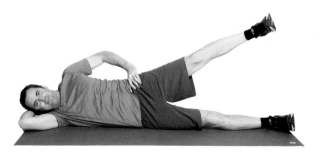

Heel dips (flat surface)

Heel dips strengthen your calves, Achilles tendons, and other muscles and connective tissue in your lower leg.

Standing on the floor, rise up on your toes. Now, put all of your weight on one foot and slowly lower the heel of that foot toward the floor. At the moment your heel touches the floor, use both feet to rise back up, then repeat. Start with 2–5 repetitions for each foot. Gradually build up to 20 repetitions for each foot. Once you've mastered heel dips on a flat surface, begin using a platform and, when ready, dumbbells (see "Heel dips," page 225).

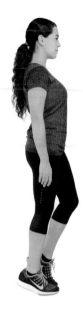

Plank

This is one of the best-known core exercises, terrific for building a stable and powerful torso.

This is basically a push-up position, except that you're resting on your elbows. Your elbows should be directly under your shoulders, and, at the other end, you should be resting on your toes. You should also have a nice straight line (or as nice as you can get) from your head to your heels. Try squeezing your glutes and tightening your abs if you feel a little wobbly. Begin by holding as long as you can maintain the position (up to a maximum of 30 seconds). Build up to one minute.

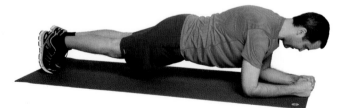

Bicycles

This is another great exercise for building your core, and it's especially beneficial for strengthening your hip flexors and quadriceps, the drivers of knee lift (good knee lift is essential for fast, fluid running).

Lie on your back with your hands behind your head and your heels slightly off the floor. Now bring one knee toward your chest, while simultaneously rotating the opposite elbow toward that knee. Don't worry if you can't touch elbow to knee; just get as close as is comfortable. Then return that leg and elbow to their starting positions as you simultaneously perform the same action with the opposite knee/elbow. Begin with 10 reps for each side, then build up (gradually, over several workouts) to a maximum of 50 reps on each side.

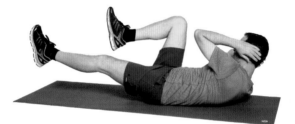

Balance on one foot

This is the simplest balance exercise of all. Beginners can wear shoes. Once you can balance on one foot for 30 seconds, try it with bare feet.

Stand straight with your knees slightly bent. Lift one foot off the floor and hold it. When you can't balance any longer, put your foot down. Do a single rep of up to 60 seconds on each side.

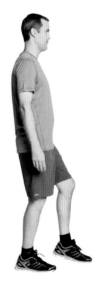

BEGINNER'S BODY STRENGTHENING — ADDITIONAL EXERCISES

The following nine exercises can be added to your routine, either in addition to the exercises you're already performing or, where noted, as replacements. You can find photo instruction for each exercise at the page indicated.

→ **Lunge walk:** See page 248.

→ **Step-downs:** See page 251.

→ **Monster walk:** See page 246.

→ **Hip adduction:** See page 237.

→ **Towel toe curls:** See page 259.

→ **Side steps (in place of ["side leg lifts"]):** See page 247.

→ **Heel dips, platform (in place of "Heel dips [flat surface]"):** See page 225.

→ **Hamstring static stretch:** See page 254.

→ **Calf static stretch:** See page 255.

ACKNOWLEDGMENTS

THE BORN AGAIN RUNNER represents more than the cathartic outpouring of a single author. Instead, it required the contributions of a talented team, all of whom have earned my heartfelt gratitude.

Thanks first to Nicholas Cizek, my editor, for his skill and guidance. And to Matthew Lore, president and publisher at The Experiment. Also to Sarah Smith, art director for the book, and to managing editor Jeanne Tao, as well as to Stuart Calderwood, the book's copy editor.

Next, thanks to my agent, Thomas Flannery Jr., and to David Vigliano and everyone else at AGI Vigliano Literary.

A huge thanks to Diana Hernandez for her photographic (and modeling) work. And to Bill Greene for allowing us to use *Sports Tutor* for multiple shoots. And to Michael P. Parkinson, PT, whose expertise informed both the injury-prevention routines and the exercise shoots.

Thanks to both Dr. Aurelia Nattiv and Dr. Paul Thompson for their terrific interviews.

The runner profiles were made possible by the candor and generosity of these runners: Hugh Campbell, Chuck Coats, Gideon Connelly, Samantha de la Vega, Eric Dixon, Mike Hutchins, Luis Palacios, Marissa Pearson, Suzanne Rybak, Greg Schnoor, Cori Shuford, and Brian Spangenberg. Thanks also to the photographers who provided snapshots of each runner: Bob Brock, Howard Fan, Alfred Higgs, Paul Nelson, Movin' Pictures, Mike Connors, REVEL Canyon City, Caroline Hollister, Tommy Chambers, Jennifer Mills, and Michael Andrew Kukuchka.

Thanks to the book's models for their patience and professionalism: Kevin Wile, Omar Naranjo, and Marie Champion.

And thanks to the various individuals, from coaches to teammates to friends, who shared my running journey, including Pat Logan, Tom McMurray, Dave Appleton, Andy DiConti, Brad Jensen, Bob Montgomery, Tom Reed, Eric Waian, Rich Burns, Steve Moreno, Dave Clingan, Ken Stone, Mary Sikkel Miller, Sumi Verbeck, Charlene Hare, Angel

Roman, Tony Young, David Olds, Kevin Paulk, Kelly Kruell, Christian Cushing-murray, and all my running mates from La Cañada High School, Glendale City College (California), Aztlán, Team Runners High, the Fluffy Bunny Track Club, Compex Racing, and the Cal Coast Track Club.

And finally, thank you to Jinny Magill and Sean Magill, who lived through so many of the times, good and bad, recounted in this book, and whose company during distance runs, drills, hill sprints, and other workouts produced my fondest memories from forty years in the sport.

INDEX

Page numbers in *italics* refer to tables and charts.

ABOUT THE AUTHOR

PETE MAGILL is a 55-year-old masters runner, coach, and writer. He is the lead author of the book *Build Your Running Body*, former senior writer and columnist for *Running Times* magazine, and former editor for *Double Runner* magazine. In his 30s, Magill was a screenwriter, with script sales to New Line Cinema and Disney. Magill has coached at the youth, high school, open, and masters levels. Over the past decade, he's led his Southern California clubs to 19 masters national championships in cross country and road racing. He's a five-time USA Masters Cross Country Runner of the Year, the fastest-ever American distance runner over age 50 in the 5K and 10K, and holds multiple American and world age-group records. Magill lives in South Pasadena, California, and competes for the Cal Coast Track Club.